28-Day Plant-Powered
HEALTH REBOOT

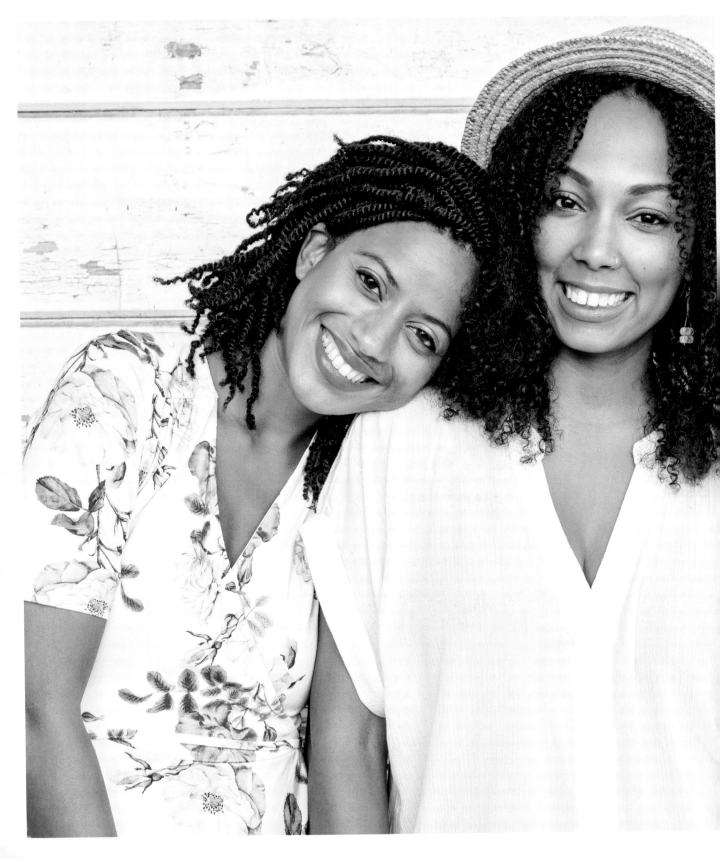

28-Day Plant-Powered
HEALTH REBOOT

RESET YOUR BODY, LOSE WEIGHT, GAIN ENERGY & FEEL GREAT

JESSICA JONES, MS, RD, CDE & **WENDY LOPEZ**, MS, RD

FOUNDERS OF THE BLOG *FOOD HEAVEN MADE EASY*

PAGE STREET
PUBLISHING CO.

PAGE STREET
PUBLISHING CO.

First published in 2017 by

Page Street Publishing Co.

27 Congress Street, Suite 105

Salem, MA 01970

www.pagestreetpublishing.com

Distributed by Macmillan; sales in Canada by The Canadian Manda Group.

20   19   18   17   1   2   3   4

ISBN-13: 978-1-62414-358-8

ISBN-10: 1-62414-358-X

Library of Congress Control Number: 2016952449

Cover and book design by Page Street Publishing Co.

Photography, food styling and propping by Toni Zernik

Printed and bound in the United States

Page Street is proud to be a member of 1% for the Planet. Members donate one percent of their sales to one or more of the over 1,500 environmental and sustainability charities across the globe who participate in this program.

DEDICATION

This book is dedicated to our followers, friends, family and clients. We've learned so much from you all. Thank you for the tremendous support throughout our journey.

TABLE OF CONTENTS

EASY LUNCH RECIPES THAT TASTE AMAZING 83

DELICIOUS DINNERS TO END YOUR DAY RIGHT 139

SNACK WISELY 194

QUENCH YOUR THIRST WITH THESE REFRESHING, HEALTHY BEVERAGES 204

Creating Healthy Habits That Last 211

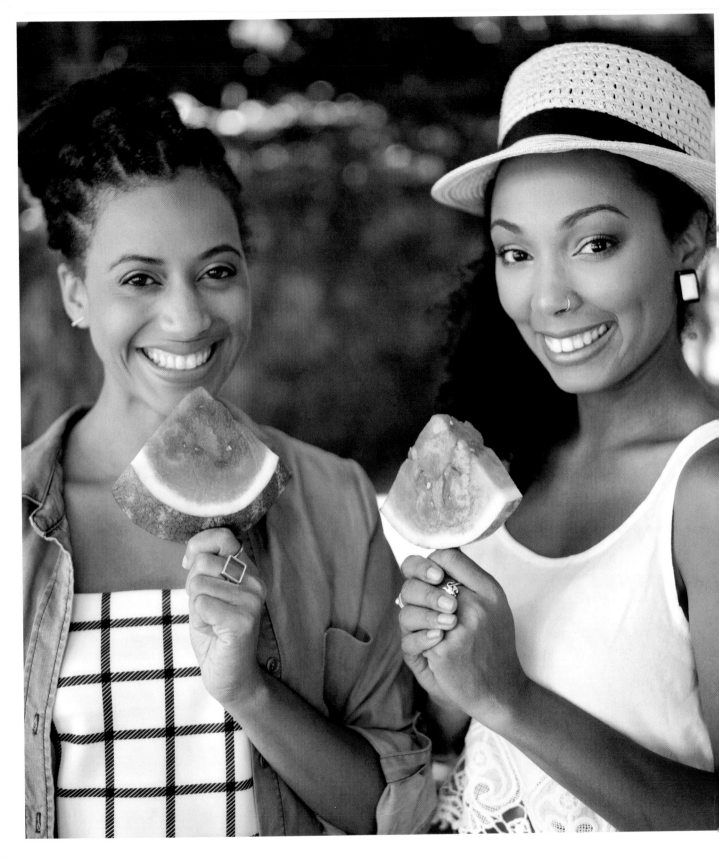

PART 1

Introduction

ABOUT THIS REBOOT

If someone were to have asked us five years ago to name our ultimate dream upon starting our healthy cooking and nutrition web series, *Food Heaven Made Easy*, it would have been to write a cookbook: A cookbook full of delicious, easy, vegetarian recipes that would debunk the myth that healthy eating is time-consuming, expensive and, frankly, gross. Although we absolutely loved the idea of writing a cookbook, having something published seemed big. Almost too big. A pipe dream that maybe would happen, one day, but not anytime soon.

And yet here we are, with a cookbook of our very own. A cookbook full of delicious, easy, vegetarian recipes. Pipe dream turned into reality? Yes, please. We've put a lot of blood, sweat and onion-induced tears into this cookbook. Our goal was to make this something that we loved. Our hope is that you love it, too.

In *28-Day Plant-Powered Health Reboot* we've created 100 recipes—all plant-powered, simple and cost-conscious. This book is perfect for those who want to become more comfortable with preparing nutritious (and delicious) vegetarian meals. Also, if you are new to the vegetarian lifestyle and want a book that helps you through the transition, this book is for you. During the first week, we give you a sample meal plan you can follow to a T (or not—it's completely up to you). Throughout the subsequent weeks, you will be the captain of the ship, deciding which recipes work best for you and how much (or little) you want to cook for the week. This plan allows you to effectively plan meals using all of our recipes, so you will be comfortable on your own after the 4 weeks are up. The beauty of this book is that you don't have to cook a completely new recipe for each meal every day. If you want to save cooking time by rotating between two to four dinner recipes throughout the week, that's fine, too—just choose recipes that have more than one serving and enjoy the leftovers throughout the week. How you structure the plan is completely up to you.

As registered dietitians, we made a point to focus on the nutrition of every single one of the recipes included here. For us, each meal needs to have the right balance of carbohydrates, fat and protein, while being under a certain number of calories (typically between 300 and 500 per serving). Within each recipe you will find the nutrition facts for each serving to help keep you on track. We also eliminated any ingredients that were not absolutely essential to the perfection of the recipe and that didn't add superior nutrition to the dish.

We want you to feel amazingly whole and nourished while completing this reboot and with minimal stress. That's why our recipes don't require 20 ingredients or obscure items that will break the bank. Who needs to spend extra money or go through the stress of creating fussy meals? Not us. Some call it minimalism; we call it Food Heaven Made Easy.

THE POWER OF PLANT-BASED EATING

Many of our readers ask us why we've adopted a vegetarian lifestyle. We became vegetarians for different reasons. For Jess, eating meat was as unpleasant as hearing nails scratching on a chalkboard. Okay, maybe not that dramatic, but almost. She never, ever, everrr, liked eating meat growing up. Fried chicken? No, thanks. Seared sirloin steak? As if. It wasn't until she was 12 years old that she learned being vegetarian was a thing, and that anyone could do it. On a family car ride home after visiting her big brother in Lake Tahoe (who at the time had a vegetarian girlfriend who introduced her to the lifestyle), she announced that she was going to become a vegetarian. That was that. She never ate meat again, and it was very easy for her to make the switch.

We realize that completely cutting out meat overnight is not a reality for most folks. For Wendy, the journey into a vegetarian lifestyle was a wee bit different. She grew up eating meat and loving every bite. Maybe a little too much. As a Dominican growing up in the Bronx, chronic illnesses—like diabetes and hypertension—were very common among her family and community members. It wasn't until she went to college that her poor nutrition started to catch up with her. She found herself in constant chronic pain with frequent, crippling bouts of constipation. As she learned more about nutrition, and began to incorporate more whole foods into her diet, she started feeling significantly better and many of her physical symptoms resolved.

Although our journeys into plant-based eating started very differently, we both agree that a plant-based way of eating is extremely important when it comes to optimizing your health and well-being—not to mention the health of your community, family members and loved ones. Notice that we said "plant-based" and not "vegetarian." That was no accident. The truth is, you do not have to be vegetarian to enjoy this cookbook or to be healthy. Shocking to hear from vegetarian dietitians, we know!

When we say "plant-based," we are referring to a diet centered around mostly whole, unrefined or minimally refined plants. It's a diet based on fruits, vegetables, nuts, seeds, whole grains and beans. This doesn't mean you have to be strictly vegan or that you have to completely eliminate meat if it is something you love. As a plant-based eater, you may want to complement meals with animal-based proteins, such as eggs, dairy, meat and seafood. The only difference is they are not the focus of your meals; instead, they are used as flavor boosters. Make sense? Keep in mind that a plant-powered diet should always be individualized based on culture, resources, religion, health needs and food preferences. It doesn't have to look the same for everyone.

There is a ton of research that suggests a plant-powered diet can help in the prevention and management of chronic illness. We've seen it time and time again with our patients. The more they include plants in their diet (mostly vegetables, but also fruits, nuts, seeds, etc.), the more they shed those extra pounds, reduce their blood sugar and lower their blood pressure and cholesterol (among countless other health benefits). Some research even suggests that plant-based eating can improve your life span. And let's not forget planet Earth. Plant-powered eating helps reduce greenhouse gases and our carbon footprint, resulting in a more sustainable environment.

GETTING THE NUTRIENTS YOU NEED

You might be wondering whether it's possible to get all of the necessary macro and micronutrients on a vegetarian diet. The answer is absolutely. A vegetarian diet can be suitable for both adults and children, as long as you have a varied and balanced food plan. For example, greens are great, but it's not the only color vegetable you want to have on your plate. Eating a balanced diet means that the fruits and vegetables you eat should be green, red, yellow, white, purple, blue and orange. (Taste the rainbow.) Eating a variety of colors means you are consuming a variety of vitamins, minerals and phytochemicals (health-promoting properties found in plant-based foods). If you are going to transition to a vegetarian (or even plant-based) lifestyle, here are seven key nutrients you must consider:

PROTEIN

Daily Recommended Intake: 0.36 grams per every pound (454 g) of body weight OR

56 grams per day for the average sedentary man / 46 grams per day for the average sedentary woman

Sources: Tempeh, soy foods, soy milk, legumes, nuts, seeds, quinoa, dairy products, eggs

Contrary to popular belief, it's actually really easy to get enough protein on a vegetarian diet. For example, the average sedentary man needs 56 grams of protein per day. This could be obtained by eating 1 ounce (28 g) almonds (6 grams protein), 1 cup (200 g) cooked lentils (18 grams), 1 cup (235 ml) soy milk (8 grams) and 1 cup (245 g) nonfat, plain Greek yogurt (24 grams). Whatever you do, try not to go overboard on all the heavily processed vegetarian "meat" products because they contain a lot of preservatives and other not-so-healthy ingredients.

FAT

Daily Recommended Intake: 20 to 35 percent of your total calories per day

Sources: ALA—Ground flaxseed, walnuts, canola oil, soy products, nuts, seeds, avocados
EPA/DHA—Fish/fish oils, specialty eggs

There are good fats, sometimes fats and horrible fats. Good fats (unsaturated) are mainly found in plants. Sometimes fats (saturated) are mainly found in animal products. Horrible fats (trans) are man-made.

Forget what you've heard. Fats are good. In fact, we absolutely need them to aid growth and development, supply energy, assist absorption of certain vitamins, provide cushioning for our organs and maintain cell membranes. Whether you are a vegetarian or meat eater, aim to consume mostly unsaturated fats, which have more beneficial health properties.

CALCIUM

Daily Recommended Intake: 1000 mg per day for adults

Sources: Almond butter, tahini, figs, soy protein, soy nuts, kale, broccoli, collards, mustard greens, corn tortillas (processed with lime), vegetarian baked beans, black beans, fortified soy milk, fortified rice milk, dairy products

We need calcium for heart function and muscle contraction as well as strong and healthy bones and teeth. However, this mineral is poorly absorbed from some beans and high-oxalate veggies, like spinach and beet greens. It's better absorbed from soy products, kale, collards, mustard greens and broccoli, so be sure to incorporate these foods into your diet. Also, having adequate vitamin D in your diet is essential, as it helps with the absorption of calcium.

VITAMIN D

Daily Recommended Intake: 600 International Units (800 for older adults) per day

Sources: Fortified soy milk, fortified cow's milk, fortified breakfast cereals, egg yolks, cod liver oil

Vitamin D is synthesized via sun exposure, so the darker your skin, the greater chance you have of melanin interfering with synthesis. Research suggests that 5 to 30 minutes of sun exposure, between 10 a.m. and 3 p.m., at least two times a week without sunscreen, should be enough for your body to make the needed amount of vitamin D. If you aren't getting sun, fish and egg yolks are among the few sources of vitamin D in foods. If you're vegan and don't get adequate sun exposure throughout the day, be sure to consume foods fortified with vitamin D. If not, supplementation is a must.

VITAMIN B$_{12}$

Daily Recommended Intake: 2.4 mcg per day

Sources: Fortified meat analogs, fortified breakfast cereals, fortified soy milk, fortified almond milk, nutritional yeast, dairy, eggs

Vitamin B$_{12}$ is the only vitamin that occurs naturally in animal products. For vegans, it's important to consume products that have been fortified with vitamin B$_{12}$, such as breakfast cereals or soy milk. If not, we recommend supplementation.

IRON

Daily Recommended Intake: Varies depending on age and if you are pregnant, but generally between 7 and 27 mg per day

Sources: Bran flakes, instant oatmeal, 100% whole-wheat bread, nuts, nut butters, potato with skin, dried fruits, legumes, fortified cereals, whole-grain cereals

There are two types of iron: heme and nonheme. Heme iron, which is found in animal products, is better absorbed by our bodies than nonheme iron, which is found in plants. Additionally, vegetarians are more likely to consume whole grains and legumes, which contain phytate, a property in some plant-based foods that inhibits the absorption of iron. To counteract this, try eating iron-rich meals with vitamin C (lemon, orange and other citrus), which enhances iron absorption. Avoid eating calcium-rich foods while eating foods high in iron, because calcium can also inhibit iron absorption.

ZINC

Daily Recommended Intake: 8 mg per day for women / 11 mg per day for men

Sources: Tofu, tempeh, whole grains, nuts, seeds, legumes, fortified breakfast cereals, dairy

As with iron, the phytate in vegetarian diets interferes with the absorption of zinc. Soaking dried beans and tossing out the water before cooking can lower the phytate content, increasing zinc absorption.

CALCULATING YOUR CALORIC NEEDS

Below is a guideline for estimating caloric needs, based on your age, sex and physical activity level. Every meal and snack in this plan comes with the exact amount of calories, carbohydrates, fat and protein to make sure you are falling within your daily ranges. Keep in mind that this estimated caloric intake is appropriate if you want to maintain your current weight. If you are looking to lose weight, you should subtract 250–500 calories from your total daily calorie needs. For example, if you are a 31-year-old sedentary woman, to maintain your weight, you would need an estimated 1800 calories per day based on this guideline. However, if you wanted to lose weight, we recommend you cut your daily intake down to 1300 to 1550 calories or increase your physical activity level. Always remember that you should never eat less than 1200 calories per day.

WOMEN			
AGE	SEDENTARY ACTIVITY LEVEL	MODERATELY ACTIVE ACTIVITY LEVEL	ACTIVE ACTIVITY LEVEL
18	1800	2000	2400
19–25	2000	2200	2400
26–30	1800	2000	2400
31–50	1800	2000	2200
51–60	1600	1800	2200
61+	1600	1800	2000

AGE	SEDENTARY ACTIVITY LEVEL	MODERATELY ACTIVE ACTIVITY LEVEL	ACTIVE ACTIVITY LEVEL
MEN			
18	2400	2800	3200
19–20	2600	2800	3000
21–25	2400	2800	3000
26–35	2400	2600	3000
36–40	2400	2600	2800
41–45	2200	2600	2800
46–55	2200	2400	2800
56–60	2200	2400	2600
61–65	2000	2400	2600
66–75	2000	2200	2600
76+	2000	2200	2400

RECOMMENDED MACRONUTRIENT RANGES

45–65% of total calories from carbohydrates

10–35% of total calories from protein

20–35% of total calories from fat

HOW TO USE THIS BOOK

The goal of this 28-day reboot is to help you support your body's natural detoxification process by learning to fuel yourself with whole, delicious, plant-based meals. This book can also be used by people who are transitioning to a vegetarian diet and are unsure where to start, and it's helpful for people who simply want to learn to cook more vegetarian/plant-based recipes.

As part of the 28-day reboot, we provide a sample meal plan for week 1 (page 24). This is because we want to start you off with structure in your quest to eat healthy plant-based meals. After the first week, we empower you to organize a meal plan that best suits your taste preferences and lifestyle using the breakfast, lunch, dinner, snack and drink recipes in the cookbook. If you are someone who needs a lot of direction, we have you covered in week 1 with an outline and grocery list for exactly what to do. And if you are someone who likes to have a bit more autonomy with meal planning, in weeks 2 through 4 you have the power to choose the breakfast, lunch, dinner and snack(s) that best suit your daily needs. After you finish the sample week 1 plan on page 24, we provide you with weekly meal-planning charts and weekly grocery shopping templates (starting on page 216) for each subsequent week. This makes it easier for you to plan (and write down!) exactly what you will be having for breakfast, lunch and dinner each day. Once you've laid out the recipes, you'll create a grocery list and go shopping.

After completing this 28-day reboot, you should feel more energized, nourished and whole. You may even lose a couple of pounds along the way (all of our recipes are super satisfying, yet calorie-controlled). You'll also have a bevy of new, healthy, creative recipes for your cooking tool kit, like Chia Banana Pancakes (page 62), Crispy Black Pepper Tofu with Green Beans (page 173), Lentil Sloppy Joes (page 108) and Spiralized Zucchini Pesto Pasta (page 162). There is absolutely something for everyone in this reboot.

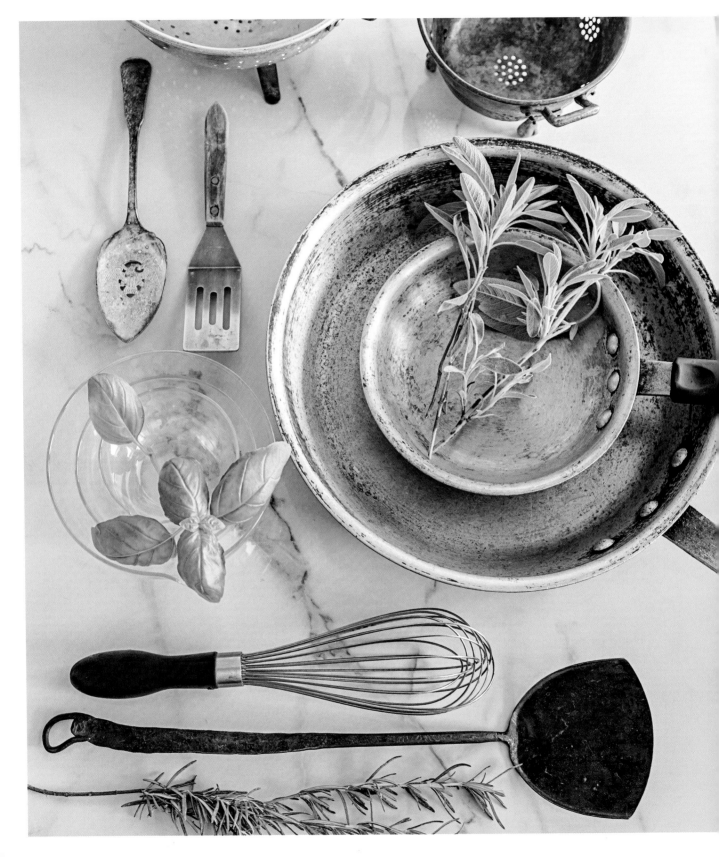

PART 2

Preparation

MEAL PLANNING MADE EASY

Meal planning is essential to healthy eating, especially when making the transition to plant-based eating. The wonderful thing about home cooking is that you control exactly what goes into your meals. As a result, you're less likely to consume high-calorie meals loaded with sodium, fat and unnecessary additives. When you have your meals prepped and ready to go, you maximize money spent on groceries and save tons of time in the kitchen. Food shopping becomes more efficient, and when going to the market, you know exactly what you'll need.

The good news is that meal planning doesn't have to be a burden—it's all about creating a setup that works for you! The first step to effective meal planning is making it a priority in your schedule. At the very minimum, dedicate 1 day per week to put your plan into action. It may be helpful to keep this meal-planning day consistent each week. Once you have chosen your day, do a food inventory. Dig into the pantry and refrigerator and find out which foods you have on hand. Aside from minimizing food waste, doing a quick inventory will give you an idea of what options you have for the week. It may be helpful to categorize your ingredients into food groups, making a list of which protein, carbohydrate, vegetable and fruit options you have.

After the inventory is done, brainstorm which meals you'll be preparing for the week. We have included a meal-planning chart on page 216, which will help you organize recipes you'll be preparing for the week. Keep in mind that for recipes that yield more than one serving, you can repurpose them throughout the week to minimize time spent cooking in the kitchen. If you find the meal plan too ambitious, just repeat your favorite recipes during the week, or make double or triple batches to cut down on time.

Once you select your meals for the week, you'll create a grocery list that includes all the ingredients you don't already have. Check out page 216 for a sample template you can use to write out your list.

SHOP THE PERIMETER

Supermarkets can be overwhelming and anxiety inducing. There are an endless amount of options, and often these options lead to confusion about what to purchase. It is helpful to map out where different food groups are within your local market. This will decrease the likelihood of wandering off and picking up items that are not on the list. The periphery of the supermarket is usually where most of the wholesome foods are stocked. Pick up your perishables first, and then go into the aisles for the rest of the items. We suggest you avoid going shopping on an empty stomach, because you'll be more likely to stray from your list and will pick up what you're craving at the moment.

Once you have your goods purchased for the week, it's time to do some pre-prep! Wash your greens, pat them dry and have them ready to go in the refrigerator. Chop onions, garlic and peppers for the week. For recipes that call for grains, cook them in batches. It's helpful to organize recipes in a way in which ingredients overlap during the week. For example, you can cook a batch of quinoa and incorporate it into the Warm Blackberry Quinoa Breakfast Bowl (page 70) and the Creamy Kale Butternut Squash Salad in a Jar (page 95).

When all your pre-prep is done, make sure you have the proper storage for your meals. Invest in containers that hold soups, salads, larger meals and sides. Doing this minimal amount of pre-prep will ease the stress of preparing and packing meals for outside the home.

7-DAY SAMPLE MEAL PLAN

If you need a little bit more guidance before fully jumping into this 28-day reboot, you'll find this 7–day sample meal plan and grocery list very helpful. We've curated a selection of recipes that pair well with each other and are relatively easy to prepare. After completing this 7–day plan, you can then use the meal planning chart on page 216 to create a meal plan of your very own using the delicious recipes in this book.

For this week, you'll be enjoying a creamy Savory Mushroom Carrot Stew (page 107), a crunchy Crispy Black Pepper Tofu with Green Beans (page 173), a simple Spiralized Zucchini Pesto Pasta (page 162), and delicious Butternut Squash Black Bean Burgers (page 193). All of our recipes have been obsessively scrutinized to make sure they hit all of our nutrition pillars: high in fiber, sufficient in protein and not excessive in calories. If something didn't quite fit the mold, we made it again, and again, and again, until we got it just right. Speaking of fiber, most of the recipes this week are loaded with it. The Creamy Kale Butternut Squash Salad in a Jar recipe (page 95) contains a hearty 12 grams of fiber. Just to put that into perspective, the daily recommended intake of fiber for women is 25 grams, and 38 grams for men. Keep in mind that as you increase your fiber intake, you will also have to increase your daily water intake. This helps move that fiber along your digestive tract to limit bloating and gastrointestinal discomfort. Aim for at least 8 cups (1.9 L) of water per day this week to complement the fiber content in these meals.

We're including a grocery list for this meal plan to make shopping a bit easier. Note that any leftover ingredients should be repurposed. These ingredients are intentionally used throughout the book so that you minimize money spent on groceries. Also note that the pantry items we suggest on page 215 are grouped together on page 21. Make sure you do a kitchen inventory to avoid buying unnecessary ingredients.

Following the grocery list, you'll find some pre-preparation tips to cut down on time and energy spent in the kitchen. Be sure to store chopped veggies in airtight containers in the refrigerator to prevent the degradation of all of those healthy vitamins and minerals.

GROCERY SHOPPING LIST

FRUITS

- [ ] 2 bananas
- [ ] 5 pitted dates
- [ ] 1 cup (148 g) blueberries
- [ ] 1 avocado
- [ ] 2 limes
- [ ] ½ lemon
- [ ] 12 black olives

VEGETABLES

- [ ] 2 cups (32 g) chopped kale
- [ ] 2 cups (40 g) arugula
- [ ] 2 cups (176 g) Brussels sprouts
- [ ] 1 small cabbage
- [ ] 1 cup (133 g) cucumber
- [ ] 7 medium carrots
- [ ] 2 red bell peppers
- [ ] 2 cups (144 g) button mushrooms
- [ ] 1 small butternut squash
- [ ] 1 medium sweet potato
- [ ] 4 tomatoes
- [ ] 2 cups (298 g) cherry tomatoes
- [ ] ½ cup (27 g) sun-dried tomatoes
- [ ] 3 medium zucchini
- [ ] 1 tsp grated fresh ginger
- [ ] 2 jalapeño peppers

- [ ] ½ cup (83 g) raw corn kernels
- [ ] 1 shallot
- [ ] 2 onions
- [ ] 3 cloves garlic
- [ ] 4 tsp (8 g) chopped scallion

HERBS

- [ ] 1 cup (60 g) parsley
- [ ] 5 mint leaves
- [ ] 2 fresh basil leaves
- [ ] 1 cup (50 g) cilantro

GRAINS

- [ ] 1½ cups (121.5 g) oatmeal or oat flour
- [ ] ¾ cup (105 g) cracked bulgur
- [ ] 1½ cups (255 g) uncooked quinoa
- [ ] 4 oz (114 g) whole-wheat spaghetti
- [ ] 2 100% whole-wheat tortillas
- [ ] 8 slices 100% whole-wheat bread
- [ ] 1 medium 100% whole-wheat roll

BEANS

- [ ] ½ cup (93 g) cooked black beans
- [ ] 1½ cups (246 g) cooked chickpeas
- [ ] 2 cups (200 g) green beans
- [ ] ¼ cup (62 g) hummus
- [ ] 1 (12-oz [340-g]) block extra-firm tofu

GROCERY SHOPPING LIST (CONTINUED)

NUTS AND SEEDS

- ☐ 3 tbsp (22 g) walnuts
- ☐ ½ cup (69 g) almonds
- ☐ ¼ cup (29 g) pumpkin seeds
- ☐ ¼ cup (60 ml) almond milk

EGGS AND DAIRY

- ☐ 1 oz (28 g) goat cheese
- ☐ 2 oz (56 g) shredded cheddar cheese
- ☐ 2 oz (56 g) mozzarella cheese
- ☐ ⅓ cup (37 g) shredded pepper Jack cheese
- ☐ ⅓ cup (82 g) plain 2% Greek yogurt
- ☐ 7 eggs
- ☐ 1 tsp unsalted butter

OTHER

- ☐ 3 tbsp (45 g) tomato paste
- ☐ 2 tbsp (16 g) cornstarch
- ☐ 2 tbsp (30 ml) soy sauce

PANTRY ITEMS

- ☐ Cayenne pepper
- ☐ Chia seeds
- ☐ Maple syrup
- ☐ Vanilla extract
- ☐ Ground cinnamon
- ☐ Baking soda
- ☐ Garlic powder
- ☐ Chili powder
- ☐ Ground cumin
- ☐ Salt
- ☐ Black pepper
- ☐ Olive oil
- ☐ Vegetable oil
- ☐ Coconut oil
- ☐ Balsamic vinegar

OPTIONAL WEEKLY PRE-PREPARATION

- ☐ Peel and chop butternut squash. Boil for 20 minutes, drain, and store in the refrigerator in an airtight container for use in Butternut Squash Black Bean Burgers (page 193) and Creamy Kale Butternut Squash Salad in a Jar (page 95).

- ☐ Wash and peel 6 carrots and boil them for 10 to 15 minutes. When cooked, drain them and store in the refrigerator in an airtight container for the Savory Mushroom Carrot Stew (page 107).

- ☐ Slice the mushrooms and store in the refrigerator in a sealed container for use in the Savory Mushroom Carrot Stew (page 107).

- ☐ If you're making oat flour from rolled oats, pulse the oats for use in the Chia Banana Pancakes (page 62) and the Hearty Oatmeal Fruit Bake (page 73). Store in a sealed container at room temperature.

- [ ] Cut the sweet potato in half and boil for 20 minutes. Drain, and store in the refrigerator in an airtight container for use in the Roasted Brussels Sprouts Goat Cheese Salad (page 96).

- [ ] Wash the Brussels sprouts, cut them in half and store in the refrigerator in a sealed container for the Roasted Brussels Sprouts Goat Cheese Salad (page 96).

- [ ] Chop the cucumber, peppers and onions. Cube the tomatoes.

- [ ] Boil 1 cup (170 g) quinoa in 2½ cups (600 ml) water for 15 to 17 minutes, for use in the Butternut Squash Black Bean Burgers (page 193), the Savory Quinoa Egg Muffins (page 42) and the Crispy Black Pepper Tofu with Green Beans (page 173). Store in the refrigerator in an airtight container.

- [ ] Boil ¾ cup (105 g) cracked bulgur in 2¼ cups (532 ml) water for 15 minutes for use in the Savory Mushroom Carrot Stew (page 107) and the Chickpea Tabbouleh (page 190). Store in the refrigerator in an airtight container.

- [ ] Cook the tofu for the Crispy Black Pepper Tofu with Green Beans (page 173) and Crispy Tofu Tortas (page 116) recipe. Remove the tofu from the package and wrap it in a clean towel. Place in a glass pan, and then put something heavy on top. The idea is to press all the water out of the tofu for up to 4 hours. Cut it into small cubes (about ½ x ½-inch [1.3 x 1.3-cm]). Oil the bottom of a baking sheet and place the cubed tofu pieces on the sheet. Bake at 375°F (190°C) for 30 minutes. Flip the tofu with a spatula halfway through so it cooks evenly. Refrigerate in an airtight container.

- [ ] Grate one-fourth of a medium zucchini for the Pepper Jack Zucchini Quesadilla (page 132) recipe. Store in an airtight container.

- [ ] Spiralize 2 medium zucchini and refrigerate in an airtight container for the Spiralized Zucchini Pesto Pasta recipe (page 162).

- [ ] If using canned beans, drain them and rinse them well under cold water to remove excess sodium. If using dried beans, check out "Beans 101" below for tips.

BEANS 101

Beans, regardless of whether they are canned or cooked from scratch, are a nutritious food that provides protein, fiber, complex carbohydrates and a range of vitamins and minerals. However, it is important to note that canned beans tend to have high levels of sodium. They may also have lower levels of key nutrients, such as vitamin A, folate, potassium and magnesium. Furthermore, canned beans cost more per serving compared to cooked beans. Does this mean you should only cook dried beans from now on? Absolutely not. Canned beans are convenient when you're pressed for time and want to whip up a quick meal. The good news is that you can use both!

With the proper planning and preparation, cooking dried beans doesn't have to be a pain. We recommend you soak the dried beans overnight in water before boiling, to cut down on the cooking time. Then drain the water, wash the beans well with cool, fresh water, and cook them in a large pot of boiling water until completely tender. Different beans require different cooking times, and cooking can take up to 1½ hours. If you have a pressure cooker, cooking time can be cut down to as little as 20 minutes. We recommend you cook a large batch, so that you can use what you need for the week. The remaining cooked beans can be frozen for up to 3 months. When ready to use, simply thaw them and add them to your recipes!

A common concern with beans is that they cause excessive gas, thanks to a nondigestible carbohydrate called oligosaccharide. To minimize discomfort, add beans gradually into your diet, and increase your intake slowly so that your body can better digest them. Also, be sure to drink plenty of water as you increase your intake of beans and other fiber-rich foods. Many of the gas-causing compounds are released into the soaking water, so change the water a few times during the soaking process. If using canned beans, rinse them well under cool water. If all else fails, you can take enzyme tablets for relief.

SAMPLE WEEK 1 MENU

DAY	BREAKFAST	LUNCH	DINNER
Day 1	Chia Banana Pancakes (page 62)	Creamy Kale Butternut Squash Salad in a Jar (page 95)	Spiralized Zucchini Pesto Pasta (page 162)
Day 2	Hearty Oatmeal Fruit Bake (page 73)	Savory Mushroom Carrot Stew (page 107)	Crispy Black Pepper Tofu with Green Beans (page 173)
Day 3	Pesto Avocado Toast (page 39)	Roasted Brussels Sprouts Goat Cheese Salad (page 96)	Butternut Squash Black Bean Burgers (page 193)
Day 4	Hearty Oatmeal Fruit Bake (page 73)	Savory Mushroom Carrot Stew (page 107)	Crispy Black Pepper Tofu with Green Beans (page 173)
Day 5	Savory Quinoa Egg Muffins (page 42)	Crispy Tofu Tortas (page 116)	Chickpea Tabbouleh (page 190)
Day 6	Hearty Oatmeal Fruit Bake (page 73)	Pepper Jack Zucchini Quesadilla (page 132)	Butternut Squash Black Bean Burgers (page 193)
Day 7	Savory Quinoa Egg Muffins (page 42)	Spiralized Zucchini Pesto Pasta (page 162)	Caprese Grilled Cheese (page 174)

Now that you're ready to meal plan like a boss, it's time to take a look at all of the mouthwatering recipes we've created and incorporate them into your week! We encourage you to customize these recipes to your liking, and bookmark any and all favorites you come across. Let's get into it!

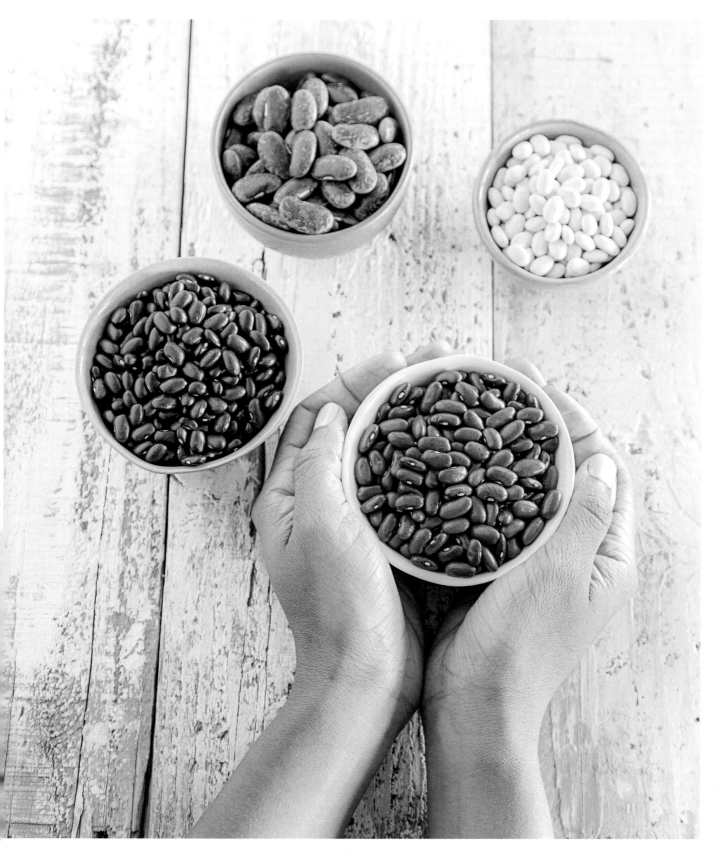

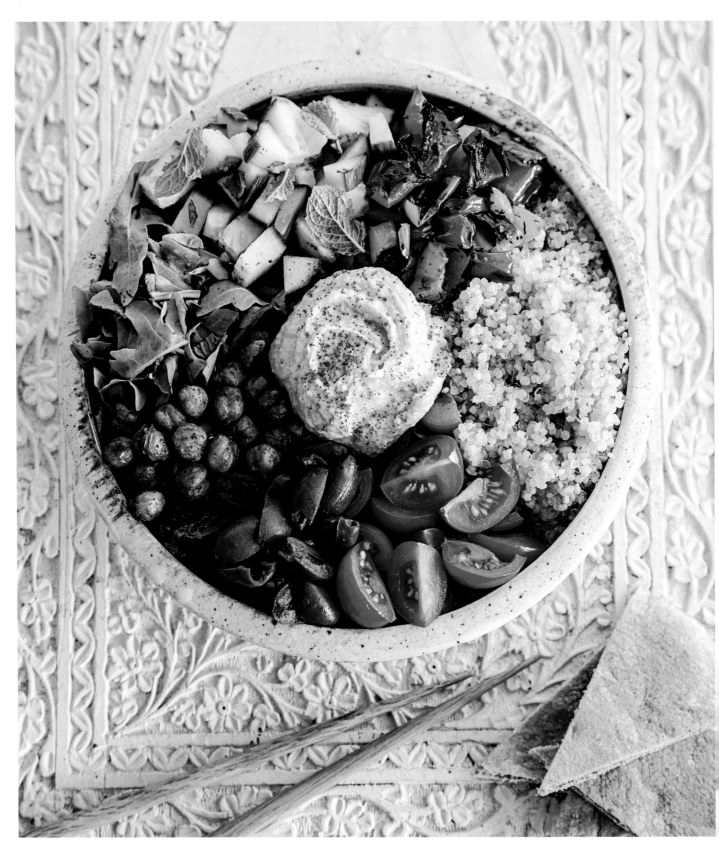

PART 3

The 28-Day Reboot: Recipes

This reboot is so simple it's a matter of picking which recipes appeal to you and planning your meals for the week. We have grouped the recipes by mealtime, but if you prefer to eat a bigger meal at lunchtime and a lighter meal at dinner, for example, then swap in what you like regardless of category. Just don't skip breakfast. Many people think that is a good way to get eating under control, but it just sends your body into starvation mode, forcing it to hold on to your fat stores in case of famine. Our breakfasts are simple yet nourishing and will keep you energized all morning. Pick ones that can be prepared the night before or in larger batches if you're in a hurry to get out the door in the morning. Remember, a nutritious breakfast will set you up for healthy, mindful eating all day, and that is the ultimate goal of this reboot.

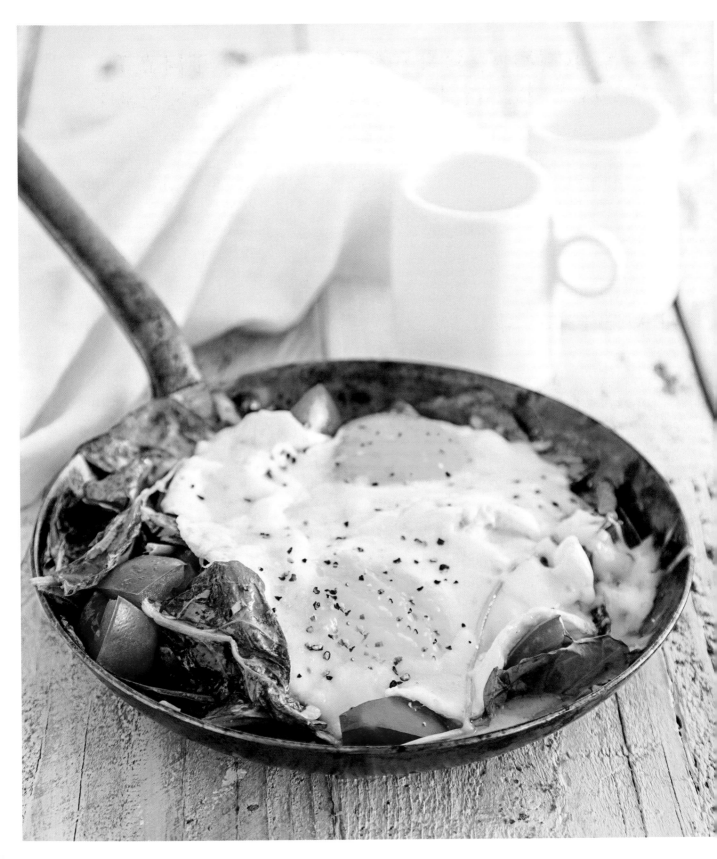

SIMPLE BREAKFASTS THAT WILL MAKE YOU FEEL GREAT

Breakfast. It's often touted as the most important meal of the day, and for good reason. The National Weight Control Registry, which tracks over 10,000 individuals who have lost weight and kept it off over time, reports that 78 percent of its members eat breakfast. Every day. We recommend that you eat a nourishing breakfast within one hour of waking up to get your day started right. Our patients find that having a healthy breakfast in the morning helps them feel great, not overeat for lunch and dinner, and reduce sugary cravings throughout the day. If you are pressed for time, try sticking to a simple breakfast, like our Creamy Chocolate Shake (page 54) or Overnight Blackberry Oatmeal Parfait (page 57). On the weekends, when you are likely to have more time to spare, enjoy our Whole-Wheat Pecan and Banana Pancakes (page 65) or Spiced Carrot Muffins (page 45).

JALAPEÑO BAKED EGGS AND SPINACH

This warm and comforting breakfast is perfect on its own or it can also be paired with your favorite breakfast side. Spinach is a nutritional powerhouse, packed with vitamin A, iron and folate. In this recipe, we'll be sautéing the spinach with onions, jalapeño and tomatoes. These ingredients, along with the eggs and cheese, work together beautifully in this one-pan meal.

Gluten-free / 30 minutes or less

Serves: 1 / **Calories:** 346 / **Carbohydrates:** 12 g / **Protein:** 21 g / **Fat:** 24 g

- 1 tsp olive oil
- ¼ medium onion, chopped
- 1 jalapeño pepper, seeded and chopped
- 1 medium tomato, cubed
- 2 cups (450 g) raw spinach
- 2 eggs
- 1 oz (28 g) shredded cheddar or mozzarella cheese
- Salt and black pepper to taste

Preheat the oven to 400°F (204°C).

Heat the olive oil in an oven-safe pan or skillet over medium heat and add the onion and jalapeño pepper. Sauté for 3 to 4 minutes, then add the cubed tomatoes. Sauté for another minute, then add the spinach to the pan. Stir for 1 minute, or until all the spinach has wilted.

Turn off the heat and crack the eggs into the pan, over the spinach. Top with shredded cheese and bake for 15 minutes. Season with salt and black pepper to taste.

SOUTHWEST SCRAMBLE WITH BAKED SWEET POTATO FRIES

These baked sweet potato fries are just as good (if not a whole lot better) than their fried counterparts. The secret is in the seasoning. We made sure to turn the flavor on full force by adding garlic powder and paprika. Sweet potatoes are a nutritional gem because one serving has about 241 percent of your vitamin A needs for the day. Studies also suggest that sweet potatoes have both antioxidant and anti-inflammatory properties. To keep the nutrition optimal, be sure to choose sweet potatoes that are firm and have no cracks, soft spots or bruises. Store in a cool, dark, well-ventilated place. We paired these sweet potatoes with a Southwest-inspired scramble because they taste great together and are nutritionally balanced. The eggs, cheese and black beans provide a powerful punch of protein, while the sweet potato is a good source of complex carbohydrates.

Gluten-free

Serves: 1 / **Calories:** 499 / **Carbohydrates:** 59 g / **Protein:** 26 g / **Fat:** 19 g

SWEET POTATO FRIES

- 1 small sweet potato
- ½ tsp vegetable oil
- 1 tsp paprika
- 1 tsp garlic powder

SOUTHWEST SCRAMBLE

- 2 eggs
- 1 tsp water
- ⅛ onion
- ¼ red bell pepper
- 1 cup (16 g) kale
- 1 tsp vegetable oil
- 1 tsp ground cumin
- ⅓ cup (61 g) cooked black beans
- ¼ cup (28 g) shredded cheddar cheese
- Salt and pepper to taste

Preheat the oven to 350°F (177°C). Line a baking sheet with parchment paper.

For the sweet potato fries, cut the sweet potatoes into sticks about ¼ inch (6 mm) to ½ inch (13 mm) wide and 3 inches (7.5 cm) long. Be sure to cut them evenly so they cook evenly. (The thinner you make them, the quicker they will cook.) Toss the sweet potatoes with the oil and sprinkle them evenly with the paprika and garlic powder. Spread the potatoes on the prepared baking sheet. Bake until the sweet potatoes are tender, about 30 minutes, flipping them once halfway through. These will come out hot, so let them cool for at least 5 minutes before serving.

For the Southwest scramble, crack the eggs into a bowl and whisk them with a fork until well blended. Add the water to the whisked eggs, as this will make them fluffier. Slice the onion and red bell pepper. Remove the stems from the kale, then chop.

Warm the oil in a skillet over medium heat and sauté the onion, pepper and kale until tender, 4 to 5 minutes. Pour in the egg mixture and let it sit for a couple of minutes, stirring occasionally. Mix the cumin with the cooked black beans and stir; then add to scramble. Top with the cheddar cheese and let the mixture sit until the cheese melts. Season with salt and pepper to taste. Serve with the fries.

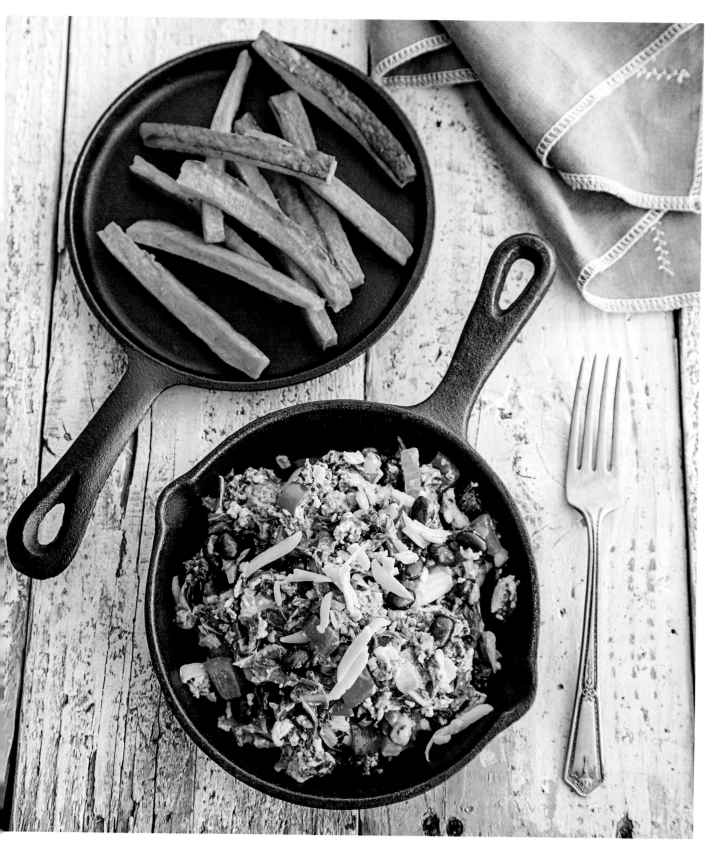

MEDITERRANEAN BREAKFAST QUESADILLAS

Mediterranean anything is pretty amazing. These breakfast quesadillas are no exception. A lot of research suggests that the Mediterranean diet might be one of the healthiest ways of eating, as the fresh vegetables, red wine and healthy fat content are thought to be cardio-protective. This recipe features one of our favorite greens—arugula—which has a spicy herbalicious taste. Arugula is technically a cruciferous vegetable and provides some of the same health benefits as broccoli, kale and Brussels sprouts.

30 minutes or less

Serves: 1 / **Calories:** 527 / **Carbohydrates:** 51 g / **Protein:** 17 g / **Fat:** 28 g

- ½ tsp olive oil
- 2 tbsp (11 g) red onion, chopped
- 2 (8" [20.5-cm]) 100% whole-wheat tortillas
- 1 oz (28 g) shredded mozzarella cheese
- ¾ cup (15 g) arugula
- 10 black olives, sliced
- 2 tbsp (31 g) feta cheese

Heat the olive oil in a pan over medium heat. Sauté the onion for 1 to 2 minutes. Remove and set aside. Warm up both tortillas in a cast-iron skillet over medium-high heat for about 15 seconds on each side.

Spread the mozzarella cheese, arugula, black olives, sautéed onion and feta cheese atop one tortilla. Then top with the second tortilla. Heat the quesadilla in the cast-iron skillet for 30 seconds on each side. You can also place the quesadilla onto a grill press and cook for 3 to 4 minutes. Cut the quesadilla into 4 pieces and enjoy the beautiful flavors this dish has to offer.

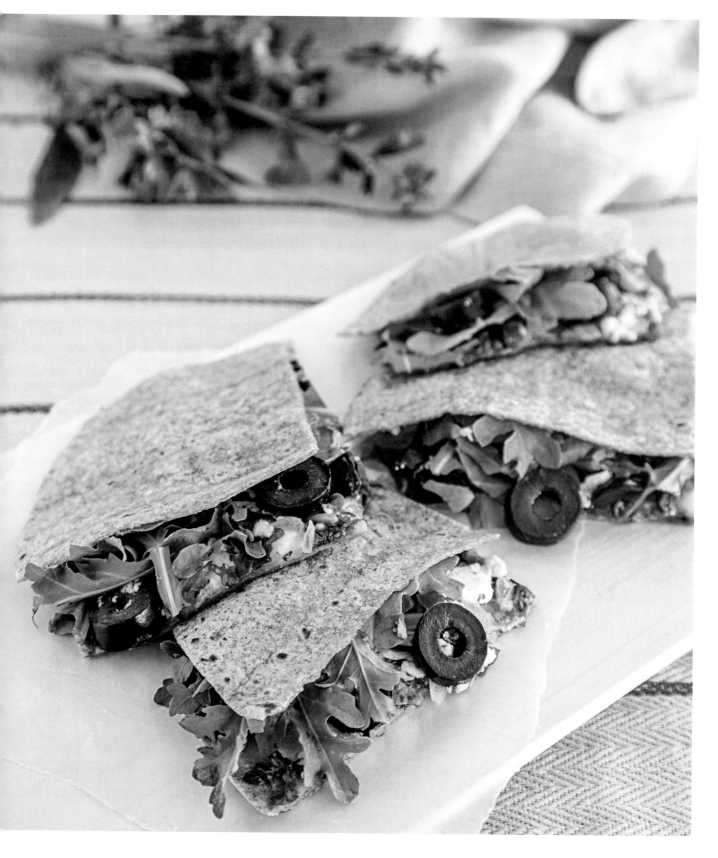

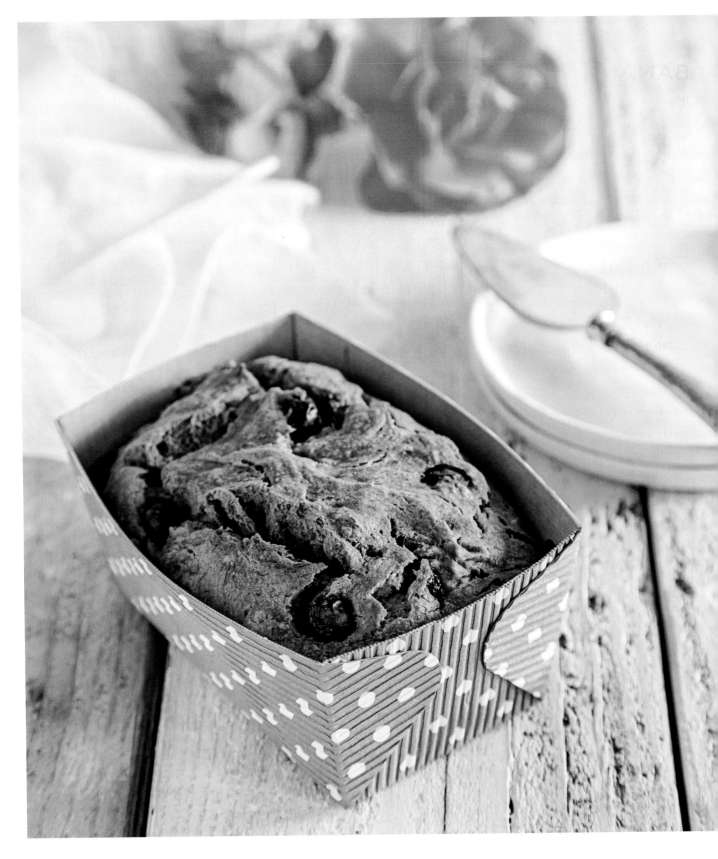

BANANA BLUEBERRY BREAD

This warm bundle of banana bread is going to add so much joy to your mornings. It's made with oat flour, which is simply made by throwing rolled oats into a blender or food processor until a flour consistency has been reached. The soluble fiber in oatmeal has been shown to help decrease LDL cholesterol and reduce the risk of heart disease. The walnuts in this recipe add a delightful crunch, while the baked blueberries literally melt in your mouth. Store leftover servings in the refrigerator and reheat for a couple of minutes when you're ready to enjoy!

Gluten-free (if using gluten-free oat flour) / Vegan

Serves: 3 (2 slices each) / **Calories:** 468 / **Carbohydrates:** 71 g / **Protein:** 8 g / **Fat:** 19 g

- 1½ cups (156 g) oat flour
- 1 tsp ground cinnamon
- ¼ cup (55 g) brown sugar
- ¾ tsp baking soda
- 2 very ripe bananas
- 1 tsp vanilla extract
- 2 tbsp (27 g) coconut oil
- 2 tbsp (30 ml) almond milk
- ¼ cup (31 g) walnuts
- ¼ cup fresh (64 g) blueberries

Preheat the oven to 350°F (177°C). Grease a mini loaf pan.

In a bowl, mix together the oat flour, cinnamon, brown sugar and baking soda. Mash the ripe bananas using a fork, and add them to the bowl, along with the vanilla extract, coconut oil and almond milk. Using a hand mixer, blend ingredients until well mixed. If you don't have a hand mixer, combine the mashed bananas, vanilla extract, coconut oil and almond milk and then add them to the bowl with the dry ingredients. Using a whisk, mix until well combined. Fold in the walnuts and blueberries, making sure they're distributed evenly in the batter.

Pour the batter into the prepared mini loaf pan. Bake for 50 minutes. It's ready when you stick a fork or toothpick through the center and it comes out clean. Remove it from the oven, and let cool for 10 minutes, then turn the loaf out of the pan and let cool completely on a wire rack.

When the banana bread is cool, cut the loaf into 6 slices. Store in the refrigerator for up to 1 week.

RICOTTA TOAST, TWO WAYS

Ricotta cheese doesn't get as much credit as it deserves. For one, its thick and creamy texture is different from other cheeses. Two, it's low in calories—only 27 calories per tablespoon (8 g). It also pairs perfectly with both savory and sweet foods. Case in point: this herbed ricotta toast breakfast paired with strawberries and sliced cucumber. This recipe is as easy as it is delicious.

30 minutes or less

Serves: 1 / **Calories:** 387 / **Carbohydrates:** 49 g / **Protein:** 17 g / **Fat:** 15 g

- 5 basil leaves, chopped
- ¼ cup (62 g) ricotta cheese
- 2 slices 100% whole-wheat bread
- ¼ cucumber, sliced
- 1 tsp olive oil
- Salt and pepper to taste
- ½ cup (83 g) sliced strawberries
- Juice of ¼ lemon

Combine the chopped basil leaves and ricotta cheese in a small bowl. Hello, herbed ricotta! Toast the whole-wheat bread, and then spread a generous amount of herbed ricotta over each slice. Top one toast with the sliced cucumber, then drizzle with olive oil and sprinkle with salt and pepper to taste. Top the other slice of toast and ricotta cheese with the sliced strawberries, then squirt with a tiny bit of lemon juice (don't add too much or it will make the toast soggy). Enjoy!

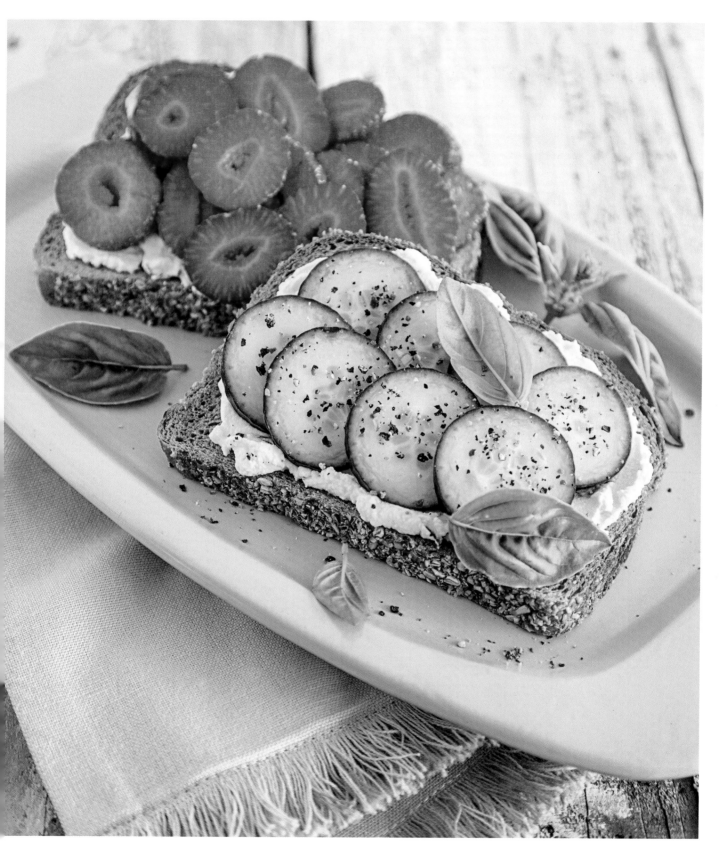

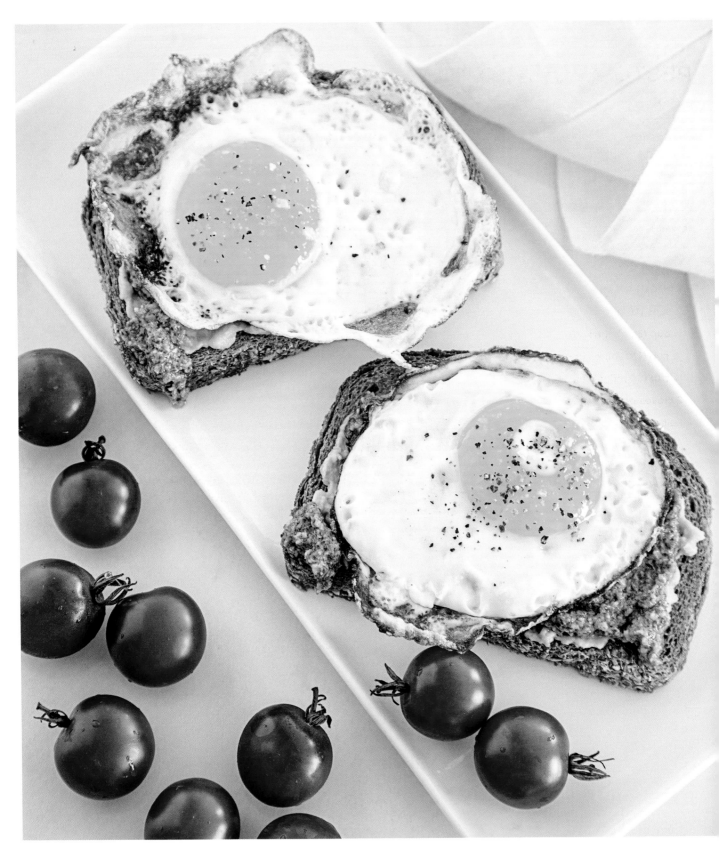

PESTO AVOCADO TOAST

By now you may have heard of the magic that is avocado toast. We literally recommend this to our patients every single day as an easy, healthy, balanced breakfast idea. Avocado toast can be done up or done simple, depending on your mood and time constraints. You could add pumpkin seeds as a topping instead of eggs, or blend in white beans with your avocado mixture to boost the protein content. With this recipe you can enjoy our simple pesto avocado toast and know that your body will feel nourished for hours.

Serves: 1 (based on 4 tsp [21 g] pesto) / **Calories:** 636 / **Carbohydrates:** 50 g / **Protein:** 24 g / **Fat:** 40 g

ARUGULA PESTO*

· 2 cups (40 g) arugula
· ¼ cup (35 g) almonds
· ½ cup (120 ml) olive oil
· ¼ cup (60 ml) water
· 2 cloves garlic
· Salt and pepper to taste

AVOCADO TOAST

· 2 slices 100% whole-wheat bread
· 1 tsp vegetable oil
· 2 eggs
· ¼ avocado
· Salt and pepper
· 10 cherry tomatoes

For the pesto, add the arugula, almonds, olive oil, water and garlic to a food processor and pulse until you get an even (but slightly chunky) consistency. Taste the pesto, and add a pinch of salt and pepper, as needed.

For the avocado toast, toast the whole-wheat bread. If you're like us and don't have a toaster (totally okay!), simply place the bread in the oven at 400°F (204°C) for 3 to 4 minutes, or until crispy but not burned. Heat the oil in a small skillet, crack the eggs into the skillet and let them cook for about 3 minutes, or until the edges are a crisp brown. Alternatively, you can cook them to your liking.

Place the avocado in a small bowl and mash it with a fork until it is somewhat creamy. Then spread half of the mash on each toast. Spread 1 to 2 teaspoons (5 to 10 g) of pesto on each slice of toast, then add mashed avocado. Top each slice with an egg and sprinkle with salt and pepper to taste. Slice the cherry tomatoes and serve on the side.

*Note
This recipe makes about 1 cup (252 g) of pesto. You will use 2 to 4 teaspoons (10 to 21 g) of pesto in this recipe and you can save the rest for other recipes, such as on pages 41 and 162. Store the pesto in an airtight container in the refrigerator for up to 1 week.

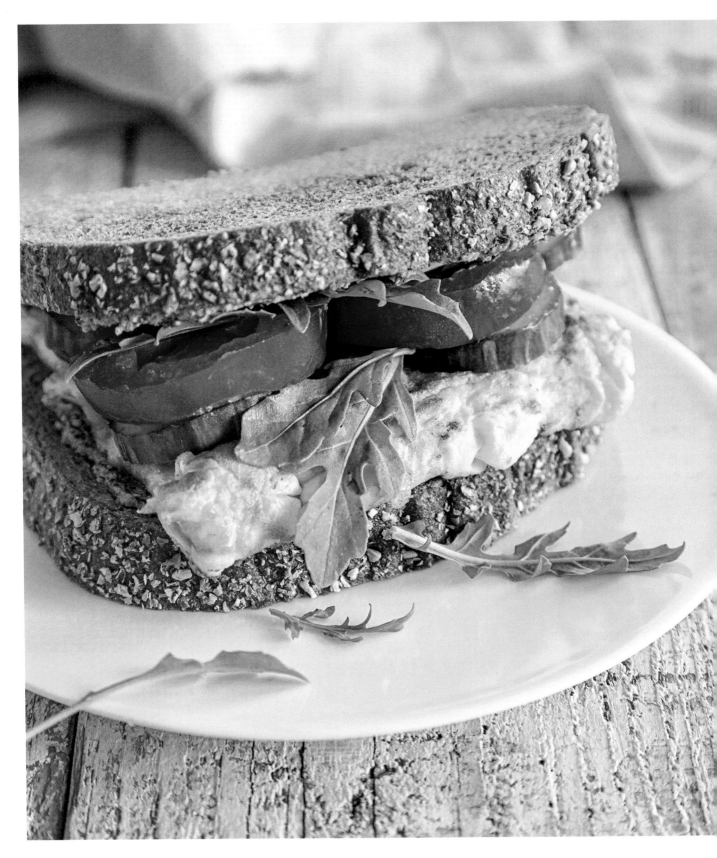

ARUGULA PESTO FLUFFY EGG SANDWICH

Eggs get such a bad rap and it's unfortunate because they are actually one of the healthiest foods on Earth. Yes, they are high in cholesterol (at about 300 mg per serving), but research suggests that dietary cholesterol (you know, the cholesterol we get from eating foods rich in it) may not raise our serum cholesterol (the cholesterol in our blood) as much as we once thought. In fact, it's estimated that in about 70 percent—or more!—of people, eating eggs will cause no increase in both total and LDL (bad) cholesterol. Enjoy this delicious pesto sandwich—and all of our egg recipes—100 percent guilt-free. If you are making this recipe as part of the week 1 meal plan, you should have leftover pesto from the Spiralized Zucchini Pesto Pasta recipe on page 162.

30 minutes or less

Serves: 1 / **Calories:** 548 / **Carbohydrates:** 44 g / **Protein:** 24 g / **Fat:** 32 g

· **2 slices 100% whole-wheat bread**

· **2 slices tomato**

· **¼ cucumber, sliced**

· **¼ cup (5 g) arugula**

· **2 eggs**

· **1 tsp water**

· **Salt and pepper to taste**

· **½ tsp vegetable oil**

· **2 tsp (10 g) Arugula Pesto (page 39)**

Toast the whole-wheat bread. If you're like us and don't have a toaster (totally okay!), simply place the bread in the oven at 400°F (204°C) for 3 to 4 minutes, or until crispy but not burned. While the bread is toasting, get your 2 slices of tomato, sliced cucumber and ¼ cup (5 g) arugula ready to go.

Beat the eggs in a bowl until well blended, then mix in the water and a pinch of salt and pepper. Heat the vegetable oil in a small nonstick skillet over medium heat. Pour in the eggs and use a heatproof rubber spatula to stir the eggs constantly to form pillowy curds (like a soft scramble). After about 2 minutes, your eggs should be mostly set, but slightly runny on top. Next, on all four sides fold the eggs toward the center of the pan, forming the perfect little square egg package. If this doesn't work for you, you can also fold the eggs in half, and then in half again.

Spread 1 teaspoon of pesto on each slice of toast, then top one slice with your fluffy eggs, tomatoes, cucumber and arugula. Top the sandwich with the other slice of bread and cut it in half. Enjoy!

SAVORY QUINOA EGG MUFFINS

These protein-rich savory egg muffins provide a wonderful range of flavors in every bite. The best part is that they're so easy to pack—just throw a couple of muffins in a container and you're all set for the morning. You can pair these with sliced avocado and/or toast for a more satisfying breakfast.

Gluten-free

Makes: 4 muffins

Per Serving (1 muffin) / **Calories:** 352 / **Carbohydrates:** 18 g / **Protein:** 22 g / **Fat:** 21 g

- ¾ cup (180 ml) water
- ¼ cup (43 g) uncooked quinoa
- Salt to taste
- 4 eggs
- 1 jalapeño pepper, seeded and finely chopped
- ¼ onion, finely chopped
- 1 small tomato, cubed
- 2 oz (57 g) shredded cheddar cheese

Preheat the oven to 350°F (177°C). We'll be using 4 cups of a standard muffin pan for baking these muffins, but you can use any size—just make sure that when you pour the batter, you only fill the muffin cup halfway. Coat the muffin cups with nonstick spray.

In a small pot, bring the water to a boil over high heat, and then add the quinoa. Lower the heat to a simmer, cover with a lid and cook for 15–17 minutes. When the quinoa is soft and fluffy, add salt to taste and allow it to cool.

While the quinoa is cooking, put the eggs, jalapeño, onion, tomato and cheddar cheese in a bowl. Whisk together well. When the quinoa has cooled, add it to the bowl with the other ingredients and, using a whisk, mix all the ingredients together.

Pour the batter halfway into your muffin cups. Bake for 20 minutes. If using a smaller muffin pan, the cooking time may be shortened. They're ready when you stick a fork or toothpick through the center and it comes out clean. Store the muffins in the refrigerator for up to 1 week.

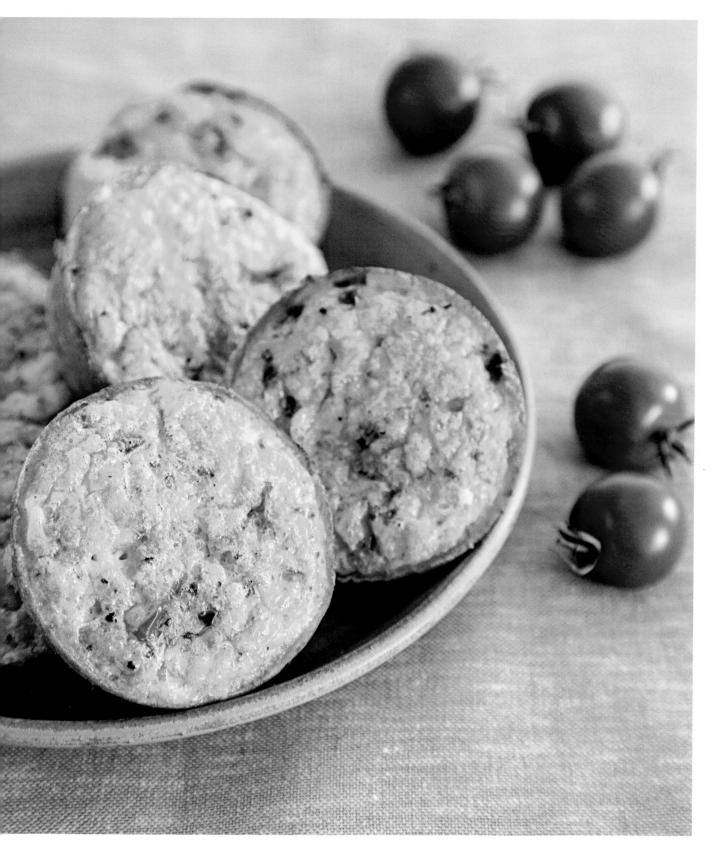

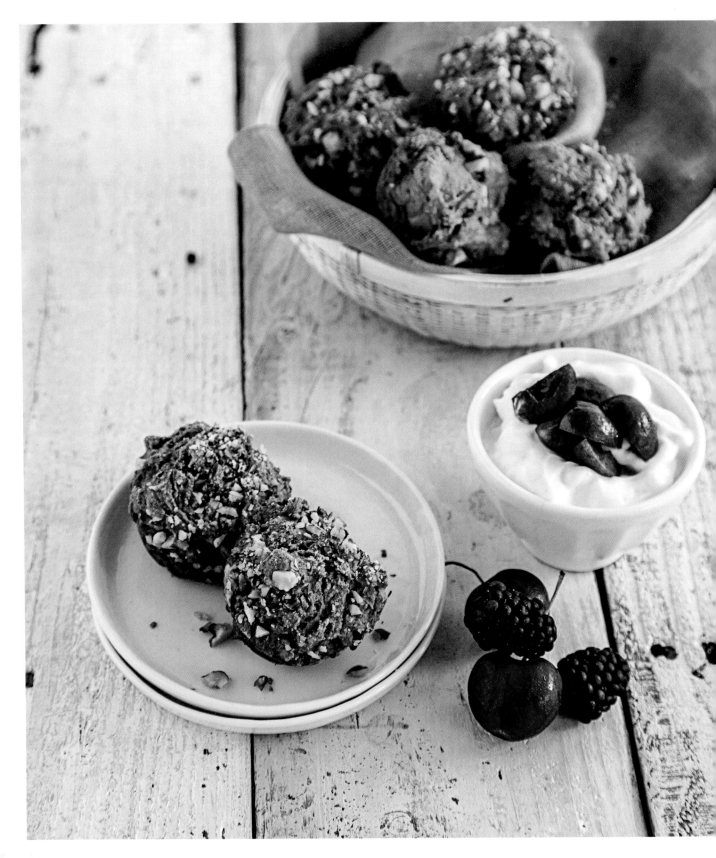

SPICED CARROT MUFFINS

These muffins add the perfect balance of moisture and sweetness to your mornings. They're packed with chopped walnuts, which add a pleasant crunch in every bite. Walnuts are the only nut with a significantly high content of omega-3 fatty acids. Incorporating them into recipes is a great way to boost your daily intake of fiber, protein and the essential minerals magnesium and phosphorus. Note that to make oat flour, you simply have to process rolled oats in a blender or food processor until they reach a flour-like consistency.

Gluten-free (if using gluten-free oats)

Makes: 3 large muffins

Per Serving (1 muffin) / **Calories:** 330 / **Carbohydrates:** 39 g / **Protein:** 11 g / **Fat:** 15 g

- ½ cup (55 g) grated carrot
- ½ ripe banana, mashed
- 1 egg
- 1 tbsp (14 g) coconut oil
- 1 tbsp (14 g) brown sugar
- ½ tsp ground cinnamon
- ½ tsp vanilla extract
- 1 tsp baking soda
- 1 cup (104 g) oat flour
- ¼ cup (31 g) chopped walnuts

OPTIONAL
- 1 cup (245 g) plain greek yogurt or 1 serving of your favorite fruit

Preheat the oven to 350°F (177°C). We'll be using a large 6-cup muffin pan for baking these muffins, but you can use any size—just make sure that when you pour the batter, you only fill the muffin cup halfway. Coat the muffin cups with nonstick spray.

Combine the carrot, mashed banana, egg, coconut oil, brown sugar, cinnamon, vanilla, baking soda and oat flour in a bowl. Using a hand mixer, mix well until you have a thick, creamy batter. (If you don't have a hand mixer, first mash the banana with a fork then mix it with the rest of the ingredients using a whisk.) Add the chopped walnuts and stir to combine.

Pour the batter into muffin cups, filling them halfway. This batter should be enough to fill 3 large muffin cups. Bake for 30 minutes. If using a smaller muffin pan, the cooking time may be shortened. They're ready when you stick a fork or toothpick through the center and it comes out clean. Let cool.

Enjoy with 1 cup (245 g) plain Greek yogurt or 1 serving of your favorite fruit for a complete and satisfying breakfast. Store in an airtight container at room temperature for up to 5 days.

MANGO GREEN SMOOTHIE BREAKFAST BOWL

This smoothie bowl is packed with all the powerful nutrients you need to jump-start your day. The mango provides a subtle sweetness, and the pumpkin and chia seeds add a crunchy finish. Many smoothie bowl recipes we've come across are heavy on the fruits and fruit juices. This smoothie bowl provides a nice balance of greens, fruit, healthy fats and protein.

The great thing about smoothie bowls is that you can customize them with your favorites. Chopped walnuts, slivered almonds and hemp seeds are among our top picks for nutritious and tasty toppings.

Gluten-free / Vegan / 30 minutes or less

Serves: 1 / **Calories:** 379 / **Carbohydrates:** 47 g / **Protein:** 16 g / **Fat:** 16 g

SMOOTHIE

· **2 cups (450 g) raw spinach**

· **½ cup (83 g) chopped mango**

· **½ ripe banana**

· **3 strawberries, hulled**

· **1 tbsp (8 g) ground flaxseed**

· **1 cup (240 ml) soy milk**

TOPPINGS

· **½ tbsp (4 g) chia seeds**

· **1 tbsp (8 g) pumpkin seeds**

· **1 tbsp (5 g) unsweetened coconut flakes**

· **1 strawberry, sliced**

For the smoothie, purée all of the ingredients in a blender until they are smooth and thick, then pour the smoothie into a bowl. Now it's time to decorate your smoothie with toppings! You can either play around with how you organize your toppings for visual appeal, or just throw them all on there.

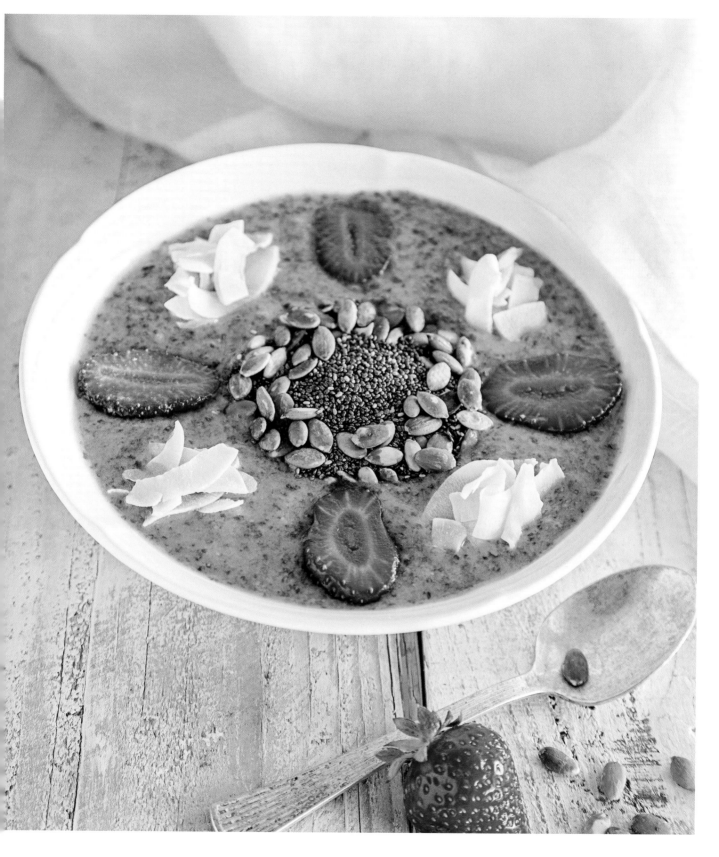

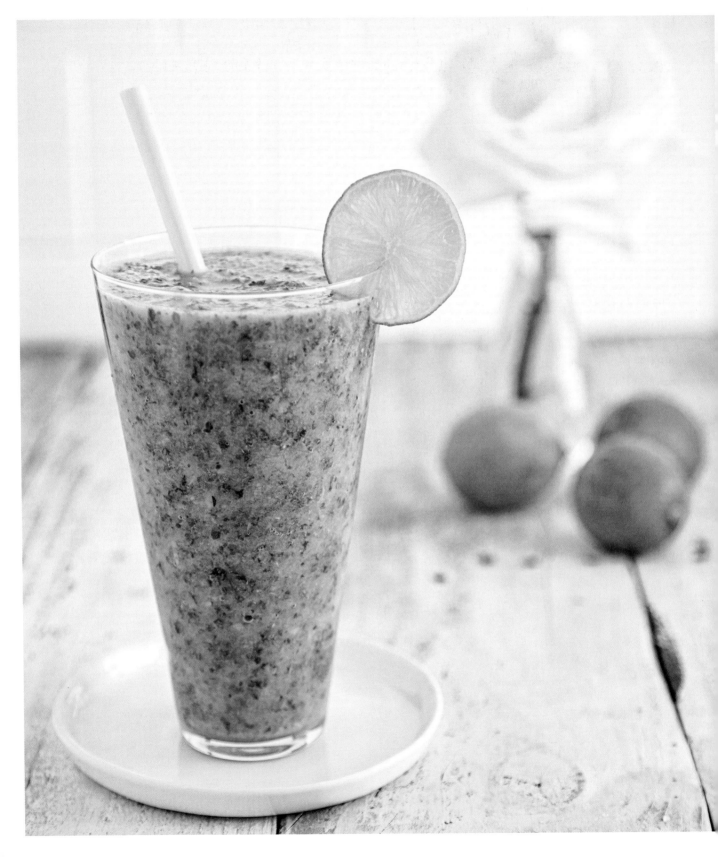

TANGY MANGO LIME BREAKFAST SMOOTHIE

This tropical smoothie is the perfect way to get your day started. Mango is one of our all-time favorite fruits. We purposely paired mango with kale in this smoothie recipe because mango helps mask the flavor of the sometimes bitter leafy green. We chose silken tofu so you get a burst of plant-based protein. Silken tofu (also called soft tofu) is a Japanese-style tofu that has a softer consistency than regular tofu, making it the perfect addition to smoothies.

Gluten-free / Vegan / 30 minutes or less

Serves: 1 / **Calories:** 330 / **Carbohydrates:** 44 g / **Protein:** 18 g / **Fat:** 11 g

- ½ cup (120 ml) water
- 1 cup (240 ml) unsweetened almond milk
- 1 cup (165 g) cubed frozen mango
- 5 oz (155 g) silken tofu
- 1 cup (16 g) kale
- 1 tsp chia seeds
- Juice of 2 limes
- 5–8 ice cubes

Add the water and almond milk to a blender (adding these ingredients first allows for better mixing). Next add the mango, tofu, kale, chia seeds and lime juice. Finally, add the ice cubes and blend until the smoothie is a creamy consistency. Depending on the strength of your blender, this usually takes 1 to 2 minutes.

STRAWBERRY BANANA BREAKFAST SMOOTHIE

Strawberries. Bananas. They're a match made in fruit heaven. We love them together in smoothies, oatmeal and pretty much any other place you can think to put them. This smoothie is perfect for a reboot because it is a great source of vegetables, fruits, protein and calcium. Have it after a morning workout for a boost of potassium to help prevent muscle soreness.

Gluten-free / 30 minutes or less

Serves: 1 / **Calories:** 420 / **Carbohydrates:** 42 g / **Protein:** 28 g / **Fat:** 17 g

- 1 cup (240 ml) unsweetened almond milk
- ½ cup (83 g) chopped strawberries
- ½ banana
- ¼ avocado
- 2 cups (450 g) raw spinach
- 1 cup (245 g) 2% Greek yogurt
- 1 tsp chia seeds
- 4–5 ice cubes
- Stevia (optional)

Add the almond milk to a blender, then add the fruits, avocado, spinach, Greek yogurt and chia seeds. Finally, add the ice cubes and blend until the smoothie is creamy. Depending on the strength of your blender, this usually takes 1 to 2 minutes. If you prefer a touch of sweetness, add stevia to taste.

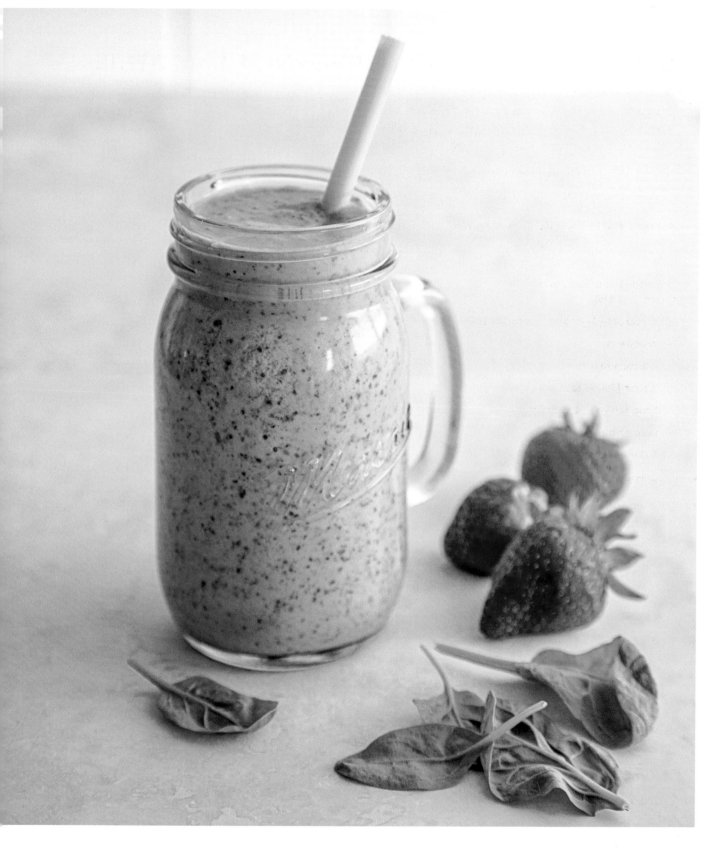

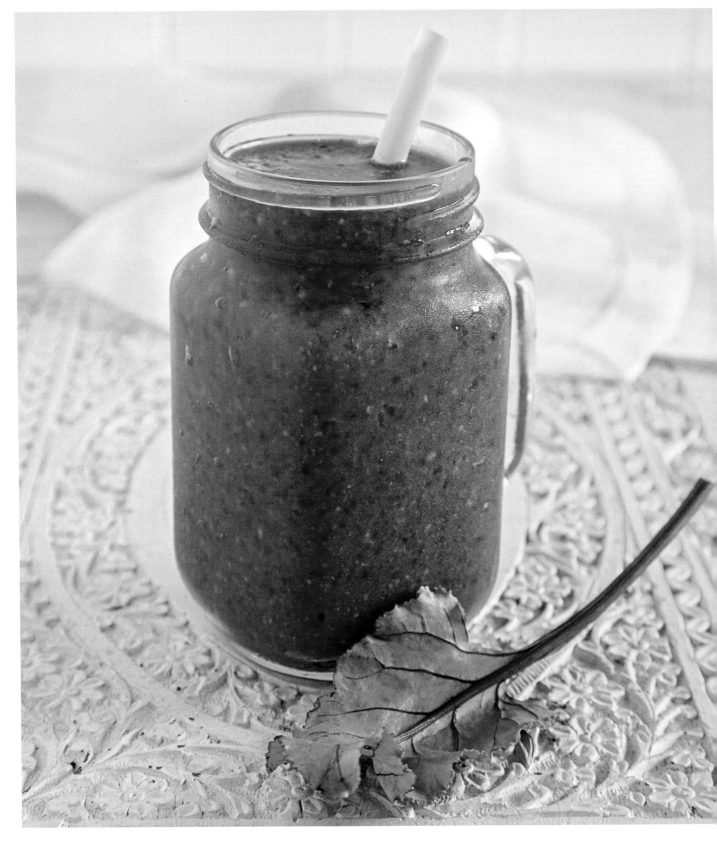

HYDRATING AVOCADO GINGER SMOOTHIE

We have a smoothie almost every morning. It's the perfect way to get a serving (or two!) of vegetables without even trying. This creamy smoothie is chock full of good fats (avocados and cashews), which will help you stay full for hours and keep your heart healthy. It also provides a dose of cinnamon, which some studies say may help regulate blood sugar levels, and ginger, which can aid digestive issues.

Gluten-free / Vegan / 30 minutes or less

Serves: 1 / **Calories:** 381 / **Carbohydrates:** 44 g / **Protein:** 8 g / **Fat:** 21 g

- 1 cup (240 ml) unsweetened almond milk
- ½ banana
- ¼ avocado
- ½ cup (67 g) chopped cucumber
- ½ beet, peeled and chopped
- ¼ cup (34 g) cashews
- 1 tsp grated fresh ginger
- ¼ tsp ground cinnamon
- 5–8 ice cubes
- Stevia (optional)

Add the almond milk to a blender, then toss in the banana, avocado, cucumber, beet, cashews, ginger and cinnamon. Finally, add the ice and blend until the smoothie is creamy. Depending on the strength of your blender, this usually takes 1 to 2 minutes. If you like your smoothie a little sweeter, add a pinch of stevia to taste.

CREAMY CHOCOLATE SHAKE

Chocolate for breakfast? Yes, we're going there. This smoothie will take less than 5 minutes to make from start to finish, so you won't have to wake up early. The beauty of this smoothie is that it tastes almost too good to be true. Think of a rich, creamy milkshake, but, well, healthy. Pure, unsweetened cocoa powder is something we ALWAYS recommend to our chocolate-loving patients because it tastes naughty but it's actually nice. This smoothie will also provide a whopping 24 grams of protein per serving, so you don't have to worry about skimping on any of the macronutrients here. Ready to blend?

Gluten-free / 30 minutes or less

Serves: 1 / **Calories:** 307 / **Carbohydrates:** 18 g / **Protein:** 24 g / **Fat:** 16 g

- 1 cup (240 ml) unsweetened vanilla-flavored almond milk
- 1 cup (245 g) 2% plain Greek yogurt
- 1½ tsp (14 g) unsweetened cocoa powder
- ⅓ avocado
- 1 tsp stevia
- 5–8 ice cubes

Add the almond milk to the blender. Then add the Greek yogurt, cocoa powder, avocado and stevia. Top with ice cubes and blend until creamy. Enjoy!

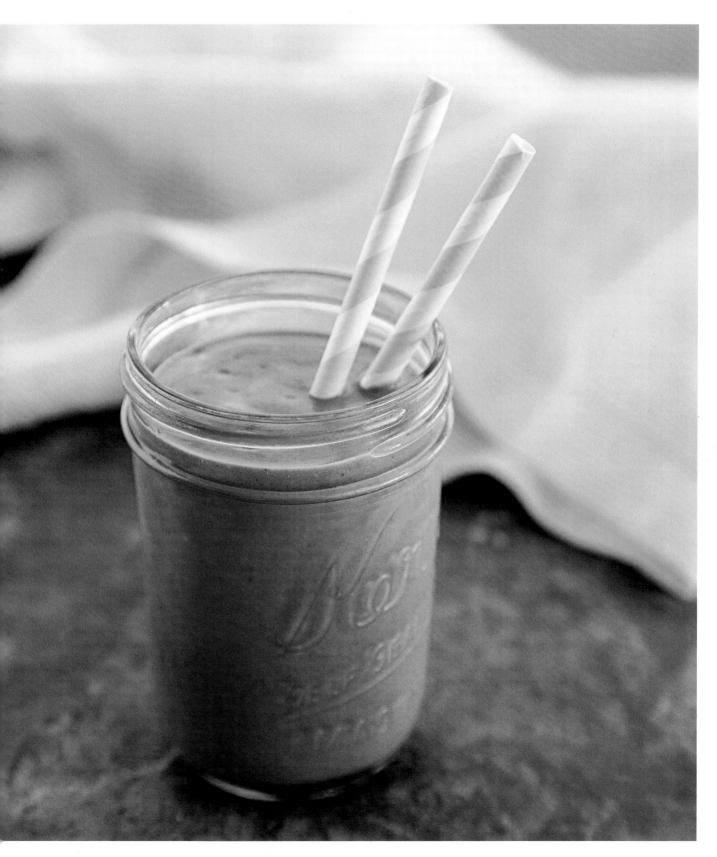

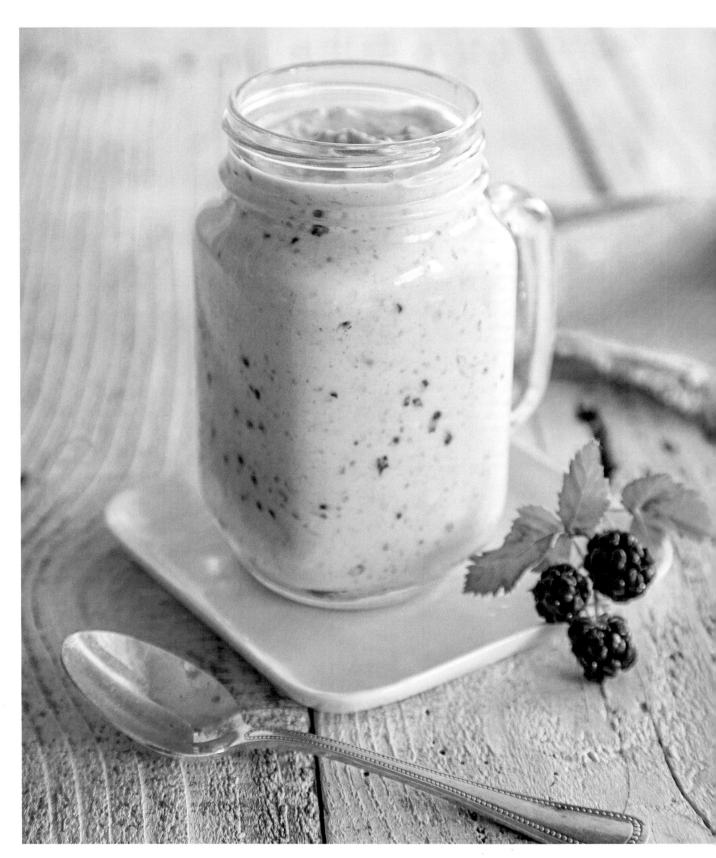

OVERNIGHT BLACKBERRY OATMEAL PARFAIT

It doesn't get any simpler than this blackberry oatmeal parfait. Just combine all of the ingredients in a jar, and let them sit overnight. The blackberries provide a beautiful purple hue to the parfait, thanks to their anthocyanins, a powerful phytonutrient that has been shown to promote health and decrease disease risk. Blackberries also happen to have one of the highest antioxidant contents among fresh fruits!

Gluten-free (if using gluten-free oats)

Serves: 1 / **Calories:** 350 / **Carbohydrates:** 47 g / **Protein:** 16 g / **Fat:** 10 g

- ½ cup (123 g) 2% Greek yogurt
- ½ cup (40 g) rolled oats
- ½ cup (120 ml) unsweetened almond milk
- ½ tsp chia seeds
- ½ cup (72 g) blackberries
- ½ tbsp (7.5 ml) maple syrup

Put all of the ingredients in a jar and mix together well with a spoon. Allow the mixture to sit overnight in the refrigerator with a lid on, or for at least 8 hours. In the morning, mix the ingredients again and puncture the blackberries with a fork, so their color can be released into the parfait. Enjoy!

STRAWBERRY BANANA OATMEAL

Warm. Cozy. Nourishing. These are words that describe this absolutely delicious breakfast dish. It's also easy to make for days when your energy is low. Balancing complex carbohydrates with healthy fats—like peanut butter—keeps your blood sugar stable and leaves you satiated until lunch.

Gluten-free (if using gluten-free oats) / Vegan / 30 minutes or less

Serves: 1 / **Calories:** 422 / **Carbohydrates:** 54 g / **Protein:** 13 g / **Fat:** 19 g
(Calculation does not include optional chia seeds)

- ½ cup (40 g) rolled oats
- 1 cup (240 ml) water
- ¼ tsp ground cinnamon
- ¼ tsp vanilla extract
- Stevia (optional)
- 2 tsp (11 g) peanut butter

- ½ cup (83 g) sliced strawberries
- ½ banana, sliced
- ¼ tsp chia seeds (optional)

Cook the oats and water according to package directions either in the microwave or on the stove. Then mix in the cinnamon and vanilla extract. Add stevia if you want it a bit sweeter. Then, mix in the peanut butter and top with the sliced strawberries and banana. Sprinkle with chia seeds if your heart desires.

PEANUT BUTTER AND CHERRY CHIA JAM OATMEAL

Did you know that jelly is made using a fruit-juice base, while jam is made by crushing the fruit? We always make jam ourselves by blending fruit with chia seeds. You'll love our peanut butter and jam oatmeal because it's delicious and healthy at the same time. In this recipe we use cherries, which contain anthocyanins, which are plant pigments that may help lower blood sugar levels in people with diabetes.

Gluten-free (if using gluten-free oats) / Vegan / 30 minutes or less

Serves: 1 / **Calories:** 350 / **Carbohydrates:** 50 g / **Protein:** 12 g / **Fat:** 12 g

- ¾ cup (115.5 g) pitted cherries
- 2 tsp (6 g) chia seeds
- Stevia (optional)
- ½ cup (40 g) rolled oats
- 1 cup (240 ml) water
- 1 tsp peanut butter

To make the chia jam, pulse the pitted cherries and chia seeds in a food processor and blend until they are a jam-like consistency. If you would like to add a little sweetness, stir in a pinch of stevia and set aside to let thicken, about 10 minutes.

Cook the oats in water according to package directions, either in the microwave or on the stove. When the oatmeal is done cooking, add the peanut butter and top with the cherry chia jam.

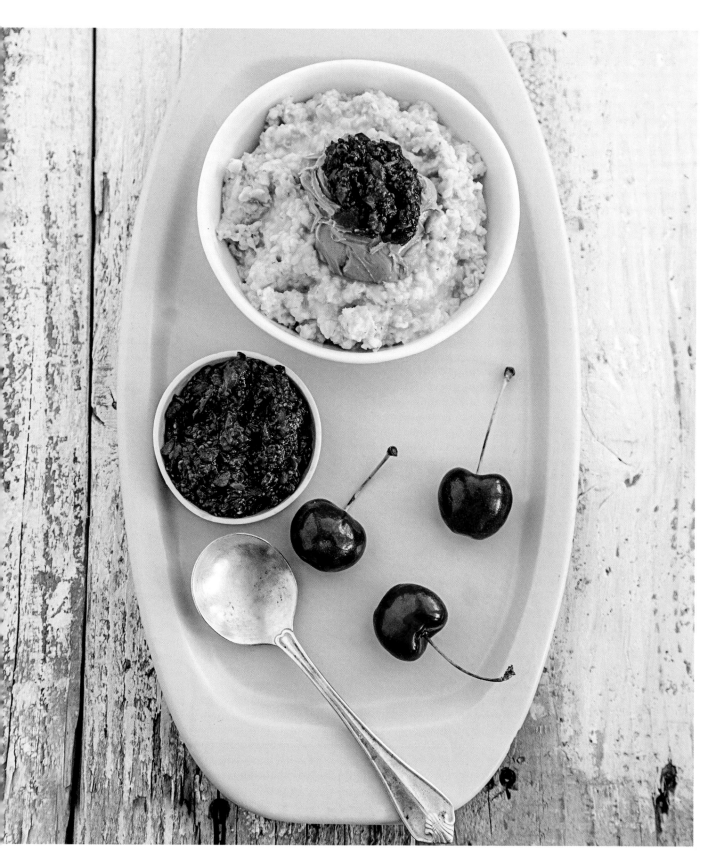

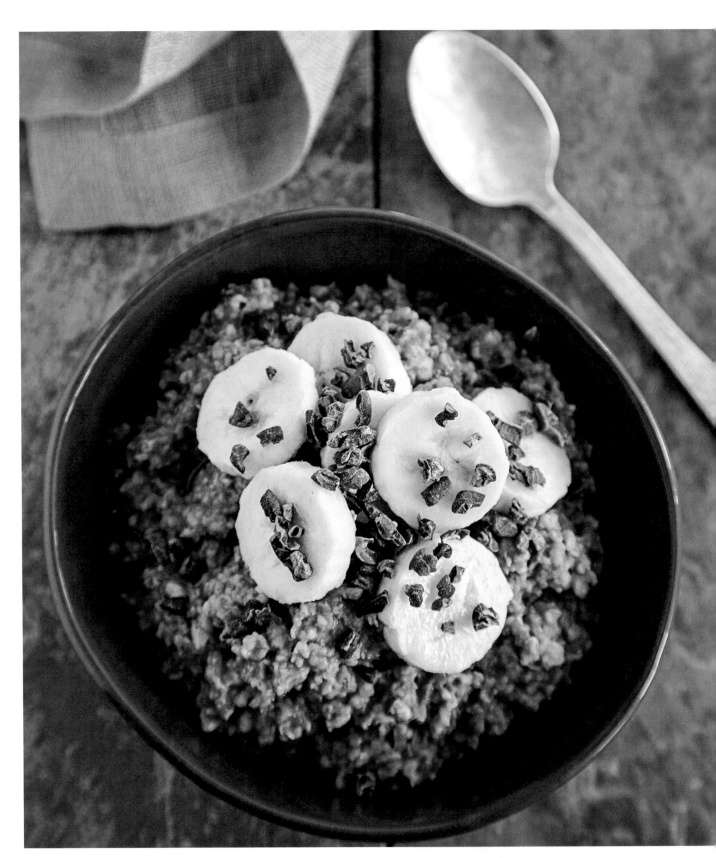

SAVORY CHOCOLATE OATMEAL

There are two types of people in this world: those who love oatmeal (Jess) and those who don't (Wendy). This recipe is so good, it can make even nonbelievers have a change of heart. The magic ingredient? Chock-oh-lah-tay. Okay . . . so forget what you may have heard. Chocolate is actually good for you. And when we say chocolate, we don't mean milk chocolate or white chocolate, which are often loaded with lots of extra ingredients (read: sugar). We're talkin' pure, dark (unsweetened) cocoa, which is a superfood powerhouse packed with antioxidants that will help your cells stay fresh and clean. If you like a good, hearty breakfast like we do (especially on those lazy weekends), then you'll love this recipe.

Gluten-free (if using gluten-free oats) / Vegan / 30 minutes or less

Serves: 1 / **Calories:** 336 / **Carbohydrates:** 61 g / **Protein:** 7 g / **Fat:** 8 g

- ½ **cup (40 g) rolled oats**
- **1 cup (240 ml) water**
- **1 tsp unsweetened cocoa powder**
- **1 tsp maple syrup**
- ½ **banana, sliced**
- **1 tsp dark chocolate cacao nibs**

Cook the oatmeal in the water according to package directions, either on the stove or in the microwave. When the oatmeal is cooked, stir in the cocoa powder. Add the maple syrup and sliced banana on top—this will also add a nice sweetness—then sprinkle with the cacao nibs and say hello to yum.

CHIA BANANA PANCAKES

Pancakes are a household favorite. We love whipping them up on a lazy Sunday, when you can relax and take your time with breakfast. Aside from adding a boost of fiber and protein, the oat flour and chia seeds work together to create a light and airy texture, which goes perfectly with the subtle sweetness of the ripe banana. Note that to make oat flour, you simply process rolled oats in a blender or food processor until they reach a flour-like consistency.

Gluten-free (if using gluten-free oats) / 30 minutes or less

Serves: 1 / **Calories:** 532 / **Carbohydrates:** 67 g / **Protein:** 17 g / **Fat:** 24 g

PANCAKES

· 1 ripe banana
· ¼ cup (26 g) oat flour
· 1 egg
· ¼ tsp baking soda
· 1 tbsp (8 g) chia seeds
· Pinch of salt

TOPPINGS

· 2 tbsp (15 g) chopped walnuts
· 1 tsp butter
· 1 tbsp (15 ml) maple syrup

To make the pancakes, add the banana, oat flour, egg, baking soda and chia seeds to a blender or food processor. Blend until smooth. Pour into a bowl and add a tiny pinch of salt. Let the batter sit for 20 minutes, so it can thicken.

Coat a pan or skillet with nonstick spray and heat over medium heat. Pour the batter into 2 medium-size pancakes and cook for 2 minutes on each side. Enjoy with the suggested toppings or customize with your own!

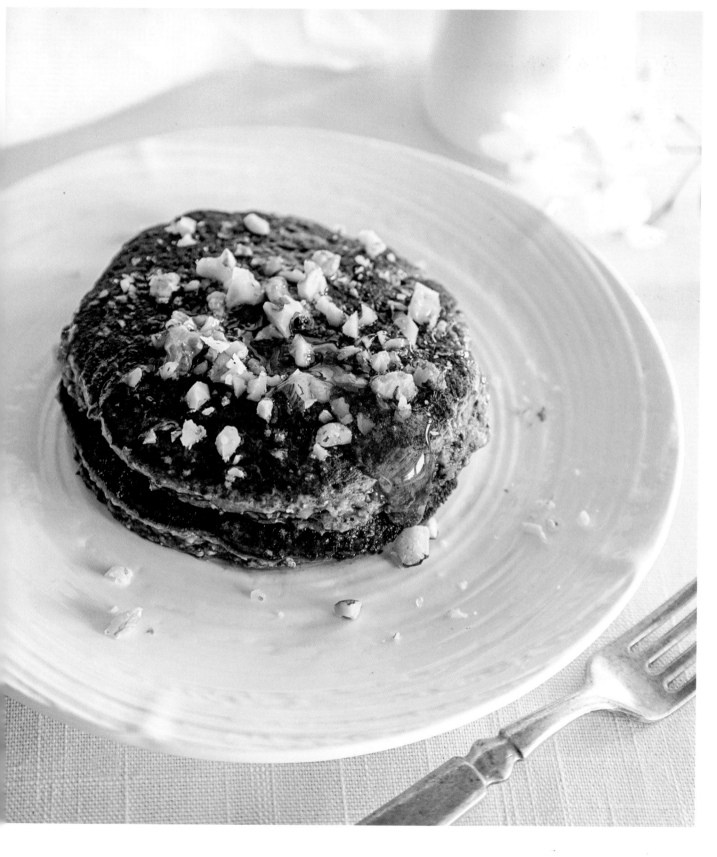

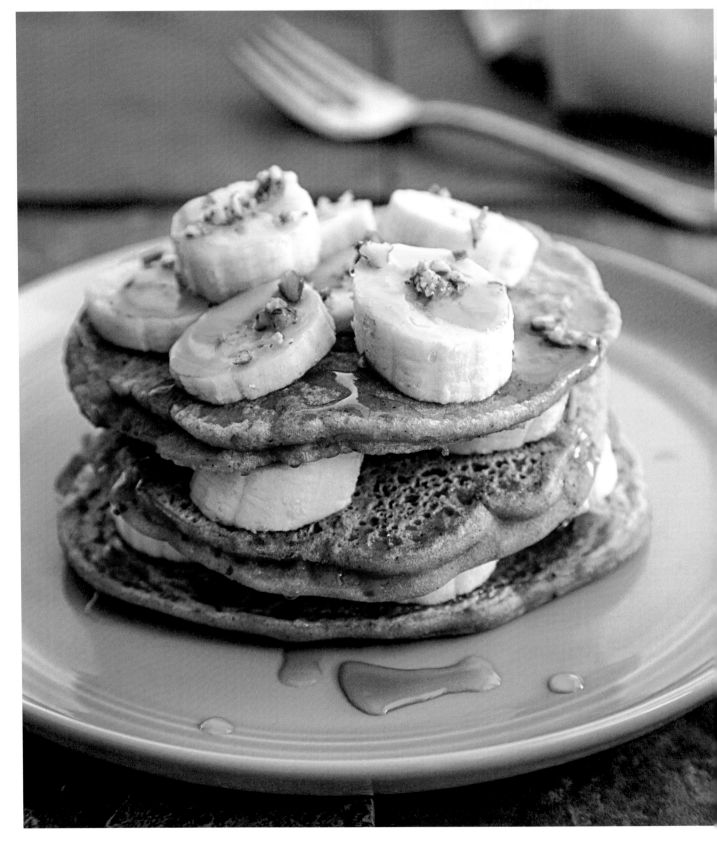

WHOLE-WHEAT PECAN AND BANANA PANCAKES

We love pancakes. (And we have never met anyone who doesn't.) These are perfect for a weekend breakfast because they are warming to the soul and will have your kitchen smelling like fall in a box. The great thing about using cinnamon and nutmeg is that you can add oodles of flavor without any health consequences. In fact, some research suggests that spices like cinnamon and nutmeg have health benefits such as blood sugar stabilization and antibacterial properties.

Vegan / 30 minutes or less

Serves: 1 / **Calories:** 671 / **Carbohydrates:** 91 g / **Protein:** 12 g / **Fat:** 29 g

- ½ cup (60 g) 100% whole-wheat flour
- ½ tsp baking soda
- 1 tsp ground cinnamon
- 1 tsp ground nutmeg
- ¾ cup (180 ml) unsweetened almond milk
- 1 tsp vegetable oil
- 2 tbsp (30 ml) maple syrup
- ½ tsp vanilla extract
- ¼ cup (55 g) pecan halves
- ½ banana, sliced

Combine the flour, baking soda, cinnamon and nutmeg in a large bowl. Add the almond milk, oil, maple syrup and vanilla and mix well until you achieve an even consistency. Toss in the pecans and mix until they are evenly dispersed throughout the batter.

Use a nonstick pan or coat your pan with cooking spray and heat over medium heat. Cook the pancakes for 2 minutes on each side. This should make about 3 pancakes. Top with the banana slices and additional syrup, if desired. We like to layer the sliced banana in between each pancake, but have fun with it!

PUMPKIN SEED AND WALNUT GRANOLA

This fiber-rich granola is the perfect balance of sweetness and crunch for your mornings. It has subtle hints of coconut and cinnamon, and the finishing touch of salt really brings together all of the flavors in this recipe. Pumpkin seeds provide fiber, protein and iron. They're also a good source of the essential minerals magnesium and zinc. For an extra boost of healthy fats, add them to smoothies, baked goods or your favorite snack recipes!

Gluten-free (if using gluten-free oats) / Vegan

Serves: 4
Per serving (granola only) **/ Calories:** 428 **/ Carbohydrates:** 43 g **/ Protein:** 9 g **/ Fat:** 26 g

- 1¾ cups (142 g) rolled oats
- ¼ cup (29 g) pumpkin seeds
- ½ cup (63 g) chopped walnuts
- ½ tsp ground cinnamon
- 2 tbsp (28 g) brown sugar
- 3 tbsp (44 ml) maple syrup
- 3 tbsp (41 g) coconut oil
- ⅛ tsp salt

Preheat the oven to 300°F (149°C). Line a large baking sheet with parchment paper.

Add the rolled oats, pumpkin seeds, chopped walnuts, cinnamon and brown sugar to a large bowl. Using your hands or a large spoon, mix well. Next, add the maple syrup and coconut oil and stir to combine well.

Scoop the granola mix onto the prepared baking sheet. Spread the granola out in a thin layer and sprinkle the salt on top. Bake for 35 minutes, flipping with a spatula after 15 minutes. The granola should be crisp and crunchy, and be a light brown color. Allow the granola to cool. Enjoy with your milk of preference or plain Greek yogurt. Store the granola in an airtight container in the refrigerator for up to 1 month.

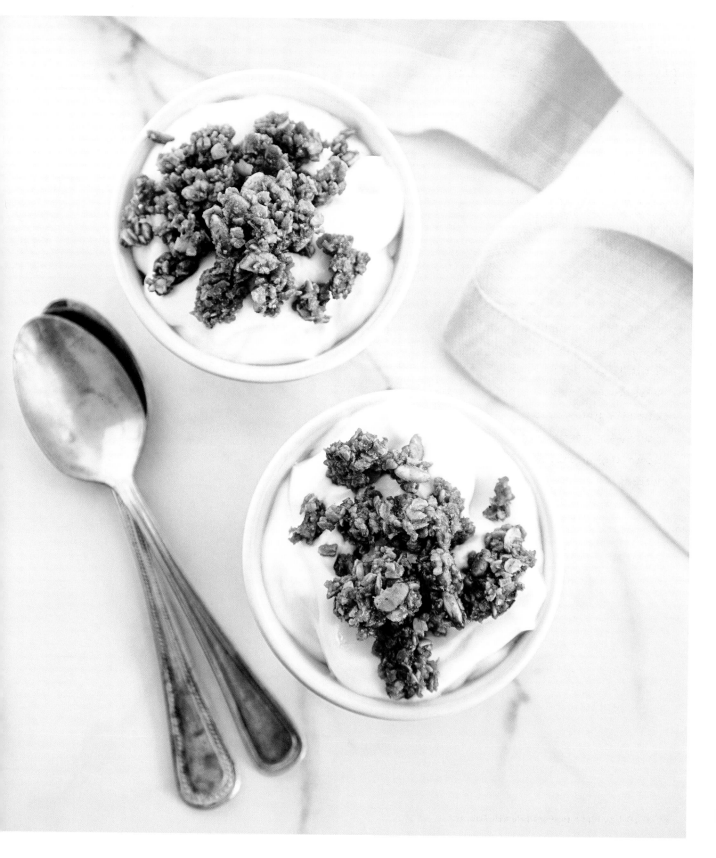

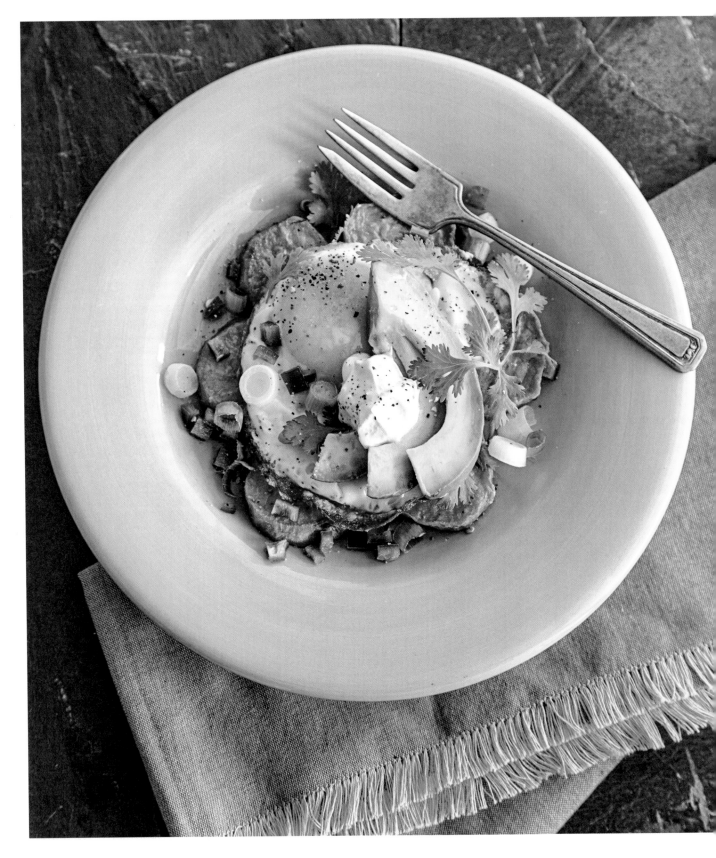

ROASTED SWEET POTATO BREAKFAST BOWL

This incredibly filling breakfast bowl is exactly what you need to boost your energy in the morning. Sweet potatoes are an excellent source of vitamins A and C. They also come packed with antioxidants, which may help reduce your risk for cancer and heart disease. In this recipe, you'll be dressing up your sweet potato bowl with cilantro, green onions, jalapeño and avocado. Need we say more?

Gluten-free

Serves: 1 / **Calories:** 390 / **Carbohydrates:** 31 g / **Protein:** 9 g / **Fat:** 25 g

- 1 small sweet potato
- 2 tsp (10 ml) coconut oil, melted, or cooking spray
- ½ tsp olive oil
- 1 egg
- ¼ cup (15 g) fresh cilantro leaves
- 2 tbsp (9 g) chopped scallion
- ½ jalapeño, seeded and chopped
- ¼ avocado
- 1 tsp sour cream
- Salt and pepper to taste

Preheat the oven to 400°F (204°C). Line a baking sheet with parchment paper.

In a medium-sized pot filled with water, boil the sweet potato for 10 minutes over medium heat. Allow the potato to cool, and then slice into ½-inch (1.3-cm) rounds. Place the rounds on the prepared baking sheet. You can either drizzle the coconut oil over the potato rounds, or use a spray to get it on uniformly. Bake for 20 minutes. Using a spatula, flip the rounds over and bake for another 5 minutes, or until the edges are crisp and browned.

While the sweet potatoes are cooking, heat the olive oil in a skillet and cook the egg your favorite way. If you want a sunny-side-up egg similar to what we have pictured here, cook over medium heat until the whites and yolk reach the desired doneness and the edges are crisp.

When the potato rounds are done, add them to a bowl, top with your cooked egg and add the fresh cilantro, scallion and jalapeño. Slice the avocado over the dish and top with the sour cream. Season with salt and pepper to taste.

WARM BLACKBERRY QUINOA BREAKFAST BOWL

This antioxidant-rich quinoa breakfast bowl will keep you satiated throughout the morning, providing close to 50 percent of your daily fiber needs! To save time, you can cook the quinoa the night before. Then, reheat it for a few minutes when you are ready to eat, and add your toppings. This breakfast also makes an excellent on-the-go option. Simply pack it into a jar or bowl and you're all set!

Gluten-free / Vegan / 30 minutes or less

Serves: 1 / **Calories:** 360 / **Carbohydrates:** 45 g / **Protein:** 13 g / **Fat:** 14 g

- 1 cup (240 ml) unsweetened almond milk
- ¼ cup (43 g) uncooked quinoa
- ½ cup (72 g) blackberries
- ½ tsp ground cinnamon
- ½ tsp vanilla extract
- 1 strawberry, sliced
- 1 tbsp (8 g) pumpkin seeds
- 1 tbsp (9 g) slivered almonds
- 1 tsp maple syrup

In a pot over low heat, bring the almond milk to a boil. Add the quinoa and let it cook with the lid on for 20 minutes, or until soft and fluffy.

While the quinoa is cooking, add the blackberries to a small bowl and, using a fork or pestle, mash them into a jam. Set aside.

When the quinoa is fully cooked, add the cinnamon and vanilla and mix in well with a spoon. Top the spiced quinoa with the mashed blackberries, sliced strawberry, pumpkin seeds and almonds. Drizzle on the maple syrup for a sweet finishing touch!

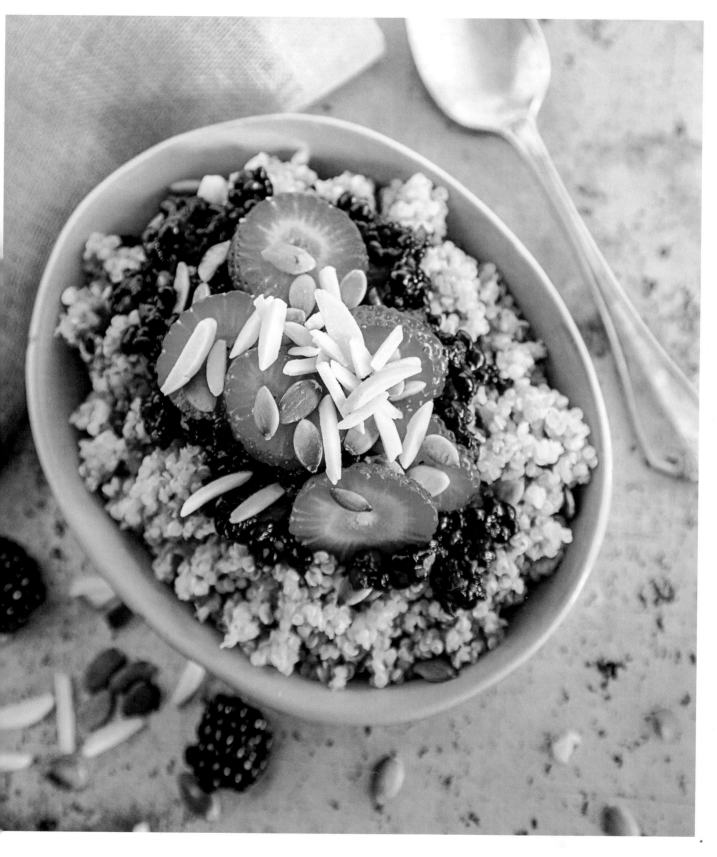

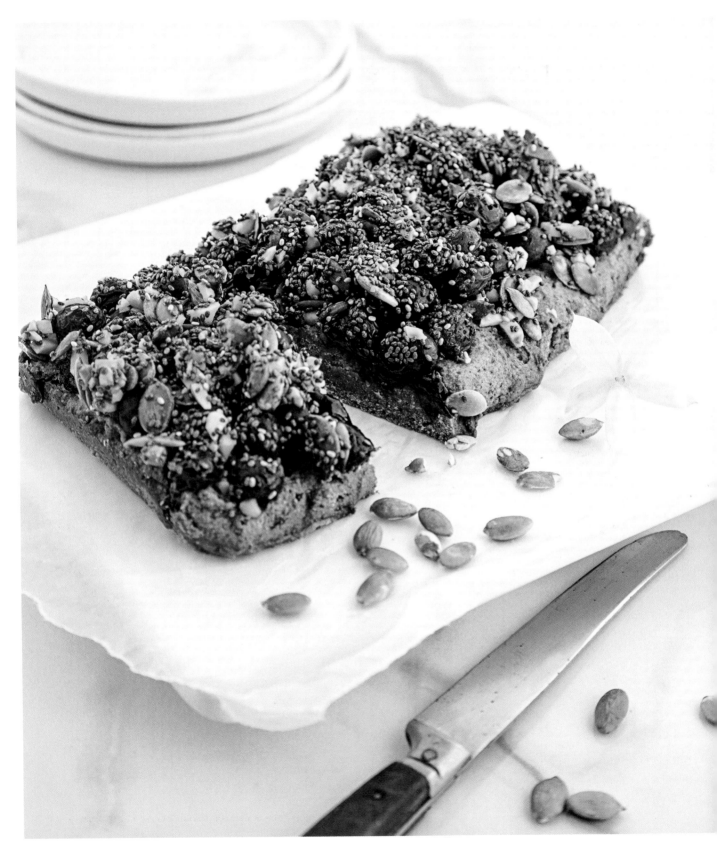

HEARTY OATMEAL FRUIT BAKE

These oatmeal breakfast bars will satisfy your sweet tooth while providing a diverse range of nutrients in each bite. Dates are used to bind the oats together and provide a savory dose of sweetness. They are a good source of fiber and are rich in polyphenols, an antioxidant that helps reduce oxidative stress in the body. The toppings also rank high on the nutrition scale. The almonds, pumpkin seeds and chia seeds will leave you feeling satisfied and ready to seize the day!

Gluten-free (if using gluten-free oat flour) / Vegan

Serves: 3

Per serving (2 squares) / **Calories:** 470 / **Carbohydrates:** 63 g / **Protein:** 14 g / **Fat:** 19 g

- **5 pitted dates**
- **1 cup (104 g) oat flour**
- **1 banana**
- **1 tbsp (14 g) coconut oil**
- **1 tsp vanilla extract**
- **1 tsp ground cinnamon**
- **1 cup (148 g) blueberries**
- **¼ cup (29 g) pumpkin seeds**
- **¼ cup (35 g) chopped or slivered almonds**
- **1 tbsp (15 ml) maple syrup**
- **1 tbsp (15 ml) almond milk**
- **1 tbsp (8 g) chia seeds**

Preheat the oven to 350°F (177°C). Line a baking sheet with parchment paper.

Soak the dates in water for at least 30 minutes, so they can soften up. When the dates are soft, put them in a food processor, along with the oat flour, banana, coconut oil, vanilla and ground cinnamon. Pulse until a firm, even paste has formed, and using your hands or a spatula, spread the paste onto the parchment paper. Using your hands, mold the paste into a 4 x 5-inch (10.25 x 13-cm) rectangle. Bake the base for 8 minutes. Remove the base from the oven and allow it to cool for a few minutes.

While the base is baking, mix together the blueberries, pumpkin seeds, almonds, maple syrup and almond milk in a bowl. The topping should have a sticky texture that will allow it to press easily onto the base. Spread the blueberry mix on the cooled base. Lightly press the ingredients into the base with your hands. Sprinkle the chia seeds on top and place back into the oven for 30 minutes or until the edges have lightly browned and hardened.

Remove from the oven and slice into 6 pieces while it is still warm. Store the slices in the refrigerator and heat it in the oven at 350°F (177°C) for 5 minutes to reheat.

CURRIED TOFU SCRAMBLE

This tofu scramble is incredibly savory and pairs beautifully with your favorite breakfast sides. Tofu is made from soybeans and is popular among vegetarians because it provides all of the essential amino acids our bodies need. It also soaks up whatever flavors you cook it in, which in this case results in a mouthwatering dish complemented by herbs and spices.

Gluten-free / Vegan / 30 minutes or less

Serves: 2

Per Serving / Calories: 280 **/ Carbohydrates:** 17 g **/ Protein:** 21 g **/ Fat:** 15 g

- ¾ (16-oz [454-g]) block firm tofu
- 1 tbsp (15 ml) olive oil
- 1 tbsp (6 g) curry powder
- ½ small onion, chopped
- ½ jalapeño pepper, seeded and chopped
- 3 cloves garlic, minced
- 2 small tomatoes, cubed
- 1 tsp smoked paprika
- ½ tsp dried oregano
- 1 tbsp (8 g) nutritional yeast
- Salt and cayenne pepper to taste

Start by pressing the excess water out of the tofu. Simply use your hands and press the tofu without having it break apart. You can also use paper towels to help press the moisture out of the tofu. Then use your hands to crumble the tofu into a bowl. Set aside.

Heat the olive oil and curry powder in a pan for 2 minutes over medium heat. Then add the chopped onion, jalapeño and minced garlic. Sauté for 3 minutes, and then add the crumbled tofu. Stir to combine, and then add the tomatoes, smoked paprika, oregano and nutritional yeast. Mix all the ingredients together well and cook over low to medium heat for 10 minutes, so the flavors can mingle. Remove from the heat and season with salt and cayenne pepper to taste. Pair with a couple of slices of toast or sliced avocado for a complete and satisfying breakfast.

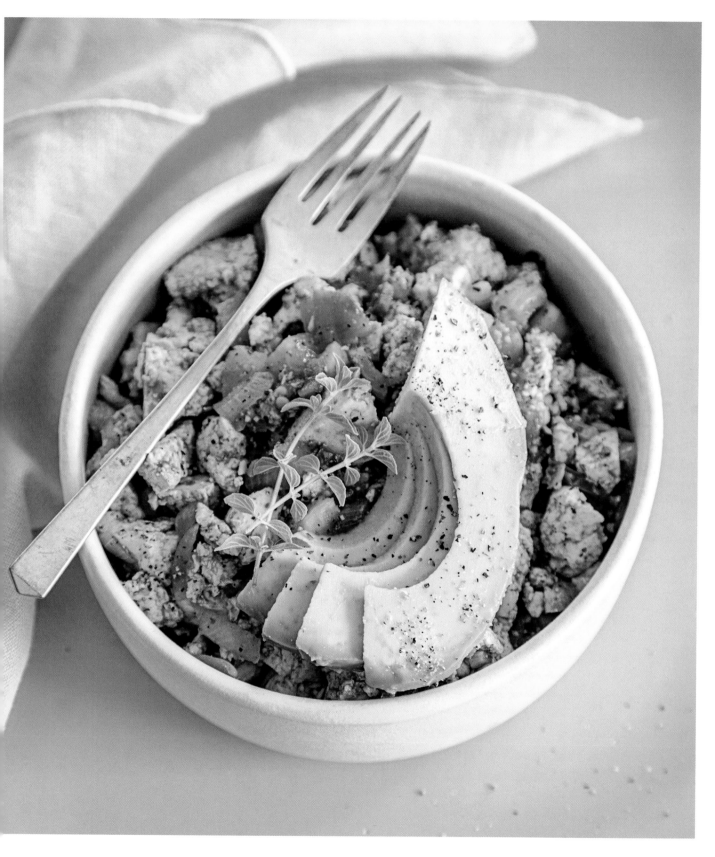

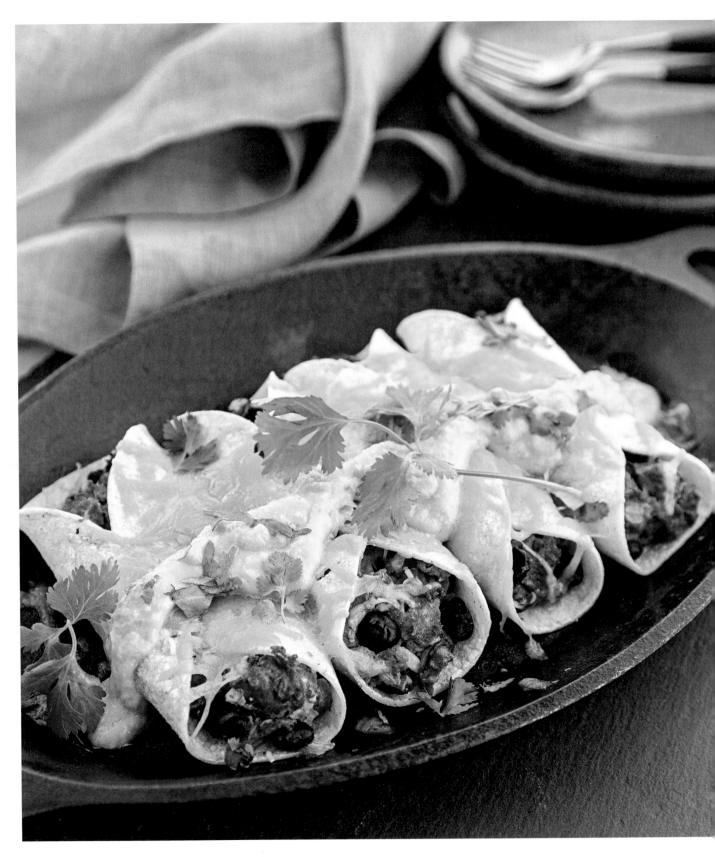

LOADED BREAKFAST ENCHILADAS

Thanks to these mouthwatering enchiladas, breakfast will never be the same. Aside from hitting the spot, this protein-packed dish will provide you with a boost of morning vitality. Black beans are valued for their protein and fiber content. They also happen to provide the essential nutrients folate, manganese and magnesium. They are one of the main ingredients for our enchilada stuffing, and you'll see how wonderfully the flavors come together after the homemade guacamole sauce is poured over the finished product!

Gluten-free / 30 minutes or less

Serves: 2
Per Serving / Calories: 466 / **Carbohydrates:** 44 g / **Protein:** 24 g / **Fat:** 24 g

· **4 eggs**

· **¼ onion, chopped**

· **½ cup (93 g) cooked black beans**

· **¼ cup (61 g) tomato sauce**

· **Salt to taste**

· **4 corn tortillas**

· **¼ cup (28 g) shredded cheddar cheese**

· **½ avocado**

· **½ small tomato, chopped**

· **½ jalapeño, seeded and chopped**

· **Juice of 1 lime**

· **2 tbsp (30 ml) water**

· **¼ cup (15 g) fresh cilantro**

Preheat the oven to 350°F (177°C).

Combine the eggs, onion, black beans and tomato sauce in a bowl. Using a whisk or a fork, beat together. Heat a nonstick pan over medium heat and add the egg mixture. Scramble for 5 minutes, until most of the eggs are cooked. Add salt to taste and set aside.

If your tortillas are not pliable, heat them for a few seconds on each side in a skillet or grill press to soften them up. Lay a tortilla on a plate. Fill the tortilla with the egg scramble, roll it up tightly, and then place it into a small baking dish or a 6-inch (15-cm) oven-safe skillet. Repeat for the remaining three tortillas. Top the rolled enchiladas with the shredded cheddar and pop into the oven for 15 minutes.

Meanwhile, add the avocado, tomato, jalapeño, lime juice and water to a blender. Blend until creamy. Pour the avocado sauce into a bowl and add salt to taste.

When the enchiladas have finished baking, pour the avocado sauce over the enchiladas and top with the fresh cilantro.

The second serving can be stored in the refrigerator for up to 1 week. To reheat, bake at 350°F (177°C) for 7 to 8 minutes or reheat in a skillet with the cover on for 10 minutes.

GOAT CHEESE AND MUSHROOM FRITTATA

This creamy and flavorful frittata recipe is as simple as can be, and the results will have you ready to make more. The mushrooms sautéed with red onion bring out a savory sweetness to the dish and the goat cheese adds a creamy and satisfying finish. Aside from being an excellent and affordable source of protein, eggs are packed with essential vitamins and minerals, and are extremely flexible in the kitchen.

Gluten-free / 30 minutes or less

Serves: 2
Per serving / Calories: 261 / **Carbohydrates:** 6 g / **Protein:** 14 g / **Fat:** 20 g

- 4 eggs
- 1 tbsp (15 ml) olive oil
- ¼ small red onion, thinly sliced
- 1 cup (72 g) sliced button mushrooms
- 1 tbsp (14 g) goat cheese
- 1 plum tomato, sliced into rounds
- Salt and pepper to taste

Preheat the oven to 400°F (204°C).

In a bowl, beat the eggs and set aside. Heat the olive oil in an oven-safe skillet over medium heat for a few seconds, and then add the sliced onion. Sauté for 2 to 3 minutes, or until golden. Add the sliced mushrooms and top with a lid. Cook for 2 minutes without stirring or mixing.

Remove the lid and add the beaten eggs to the skillet. Cook for 2 minutes and then slightly scramble everything together for 1 to 2 minutes, leaving most of the eggs in the skillet uncooked. Turn off the heat and crumble the goat cheese over the semi-raw egg mix. Top with the sliced tomato rounds. Transfer to the oven and bake for 12 to 15 minutes, or until the bottom sets and the edges are browned. Season with salt and pepper to taste and enjoy with a couple of slices of toast or sliced avocado for a satisfying breakfast!

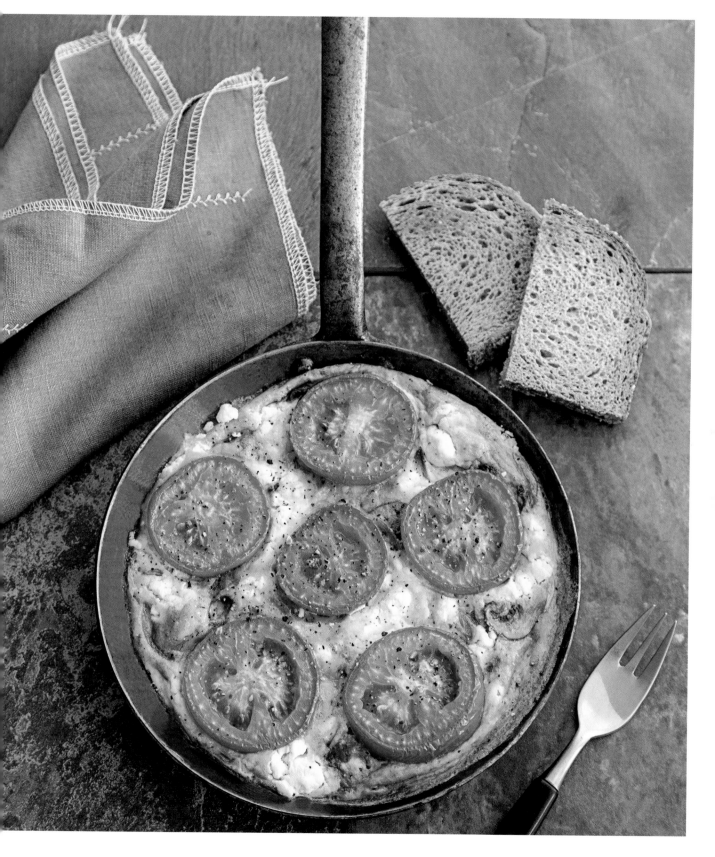

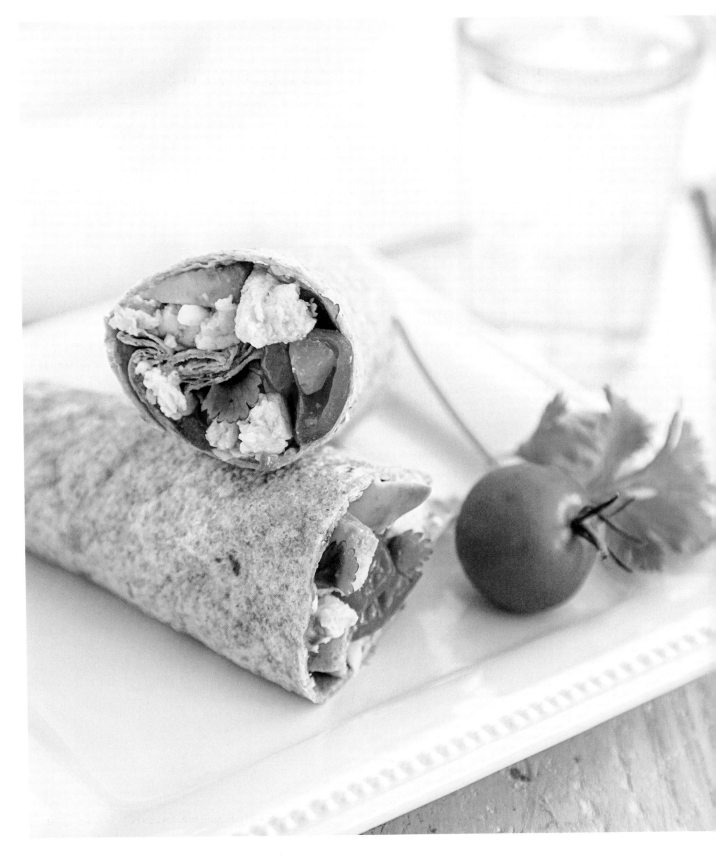

EGG AND AVOCADO BREAKFAST BURRITO

Nothing can help you welcome the morning better than a good ol' breakfast burrito. We love making this recipe first thing in the a.m. because it is super filling, delicious and takes only minutes to prepare. The pepper Jack cheese is typically flavored with sweet peppers, rosemary, habañero chiles, garlic and spicy jalapeños. We use a double dose of cilantro in this recipe to complement the Mexican flavors of the pepper Jack. Cilantro has traditionally been referred to as an "anti-diabetic" plant. In India, some regions use it to reduce inflammation. Although more research is needed, one thing's for sure—cilantro is going to kick up the flavor wherever it's included in a dish.

30 minutes or less

Serves: 1 / **Calories:** 454 / **Carbohydrates:** 43 g / **Protein:** 25 g / **Fat:** 30 g

- 2 eggs
- 1 tsp water
- ¼ tsp vegetable oil
- 1 (10" [25-cm]) 100% whole-wheat tortilla
- ¼ avocado, sliced
- ¼ cup (28 g) shredded pepper Jack cheese
- ¼ cup (15 g) chopped cilantro
- 5 cherry tomatoes, chopped

Crack the eggs into a bowl and whisk until mixed well. Add the water (this makes the eggs fluffier) and mix again. Heat the oil in a nonstick skillet over medium-low heat. Pour in the whisked eggs and let settle for about 90 seconds then begin to scramble the eggs with a spatula. The key to good eggs is to scramble them over low heat and not overcook them. As soon as they start to look fluffy, transfer them to a plate so they don't continue to cook.

Place the tortilla in the pan over medium heat, and heat for 15 to 30 seconds on each side. Watch the tortilla carefully. It should be warm, but not crispy, which is a fine line. Remove the tortilla from the pan and layer the sliced avocado on one side of the tortilla. Add the eggs, pepper Jack, cilantro and tomatoes close to the center of the burrito. Lift up the edge closest to you and wrap it firmly over the filling. Fold in the two shorter edges and keep rolling until you have a nice burrito shape.

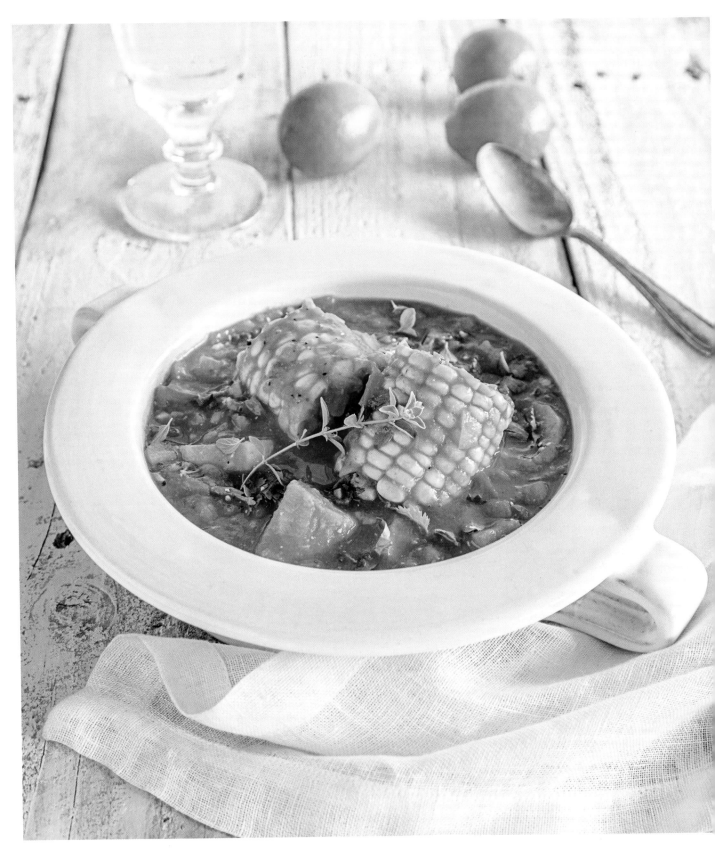

EASY LUNCH RECIPES THAT TASTE AMAZING

Eating a healthy lunch every day doesn't have to be hard. It does, however, need to be planned. If you are someone who doesn't have a lot of time, we recommend that you keep it simple by preparing just two or three of these lunch recipes throughout the week. For example, the Roasted Red Pepper Coconut Cauliflower (page 124) yields three servings. If you make that once, you can enjoy it on Monday, Tuesday and Wednesday for lunch at work. To cover Thursday and Friday, whip up something like our mouthwatering Mushroom Black Bean Enchiladas (page 123), which makes two servings. On the weekends, when you are likely to have more time, make some of our one-serving favorites, like the deliciously simple Vegan Avocado Sweet Potato Quesadilla (page 119).

VEGETARIAN SANCOCHO

In the Dominican Republic, sancocho is a thick and hearty soup made with meats, root vegetables and spices and served on special occasions. You may be thinking—sancocho with no meat? Rest assured. This recipe has been tested by a Dominican mother who specializes in sancocho, and it got two thumbs up! We use yucca and yautia, two root vegetables that can usually be found in Caribbean markets.

Gluten-free / Vegan

Serves: 2

Per serving / Calories: 474 / **Carbohydrates:** 87 g / **Protein:** 17 g / **Fat:** 8 g

- ½ cup (96 g) dried red lentils
- 1 tbsp (15 ml) olive oil
- ¼ small onion, chopped
- ½ medium red bell pepper, chopped
- 3 cloves garlic, minced
- 1 tbsp (17 g) tomato paste
- 4 cups (946 ml) water
- ½ yucca, peeled and cut in half
- ½ yautia, peeled and cut in half
- ½ medium corncob, cut in half
- ½ small green plantain, peeled and cut in half
- ¼ cup (15 g) fresh cilantro
- ½ tsp ground oregano
- Juice of ¼ lime
- Salt to taste

Boil the lentils in a pot filled with water for about 20 minutes, or until tender. Drain, cool and transfer them to a blender. Blend to a smooth puree. Set aside.

In a large pot, heat the olive oil and add the onion, red bell pepper, garlic and tomato paste. Sauté for 1 to 2 minutes, and then add the lentil purée, water, yucca, yautia, corn and plantain. Cook for 35 minutes over medium heat with the lid on, making sure to stir every 10 minutes. By the end of the cooking time, the stew should be thick and you should be able to stick a fork through the root vegetables. Stir in the fresh cilantro, ground oregano, lime juice and salt to taste.

ONE-POT CURRY RISOTTO

One-pot dishes are an absolute favorite! Just throw everything into a pot, cross your fingers and hope for the best. Well, the best is definitely what happens here. This creamy curry risotto is made with brown rice and chickpeas, which create a satisfying and well-balanced dish. The warm flavors of curry, cayenne and coconut milk complement all of the other ingredients beautifully. Everything comes together to create a rich, hearty bowl of risotto heaven.

Gluten-free (if using gluten-free soy sauce) / Vegan

Serves: 3
Per Serving / Calories: 436 / **Carbohydrates:** 42 g / **Protein:** 9 g / **Fat:** 24 g

- 1 tbsp (14 g) coconut oil
- ¼ onion, chopped
- 4 cloves garlic, minced
- ¼ cup (37 g) red bell pepper, chopped
- 3 cups (710 ml) water
- 1 cup (240 ml) coconut milk
- 1 cup (128 g) chopped carrots
- 1 cup (190 g) uncooked brown rice
- 1 cup (164 g) cooked chickpeas
- 1 tbsp (10 ml) soy sauce
- 1 tsp curry powder
- Salt and cayenne pepper to taste
- 1 cup (50 g) fresh cilantro

Heat the coconut oil in a medium-large pot over medium heat. Add the onion, garlic and chopped pepper and sauté for 3 minutes. Then add the water, coconut milk, carrots, brown rice, chickpeas, soy sauce and curry powder.

Cook over medium heat, with the lid on, for 30 minutes. Stir occasionally. Then remove the lid and cook for another 20 minutes, to allow some of the water to evaporate. Again, stir occasionally. Cook for the last 5 to 7 minutes with the lid on, taste the rice to make sure it's tender and remove from heat. Season with salt and cayenne pepper to taste and top with the fresh cilantro.

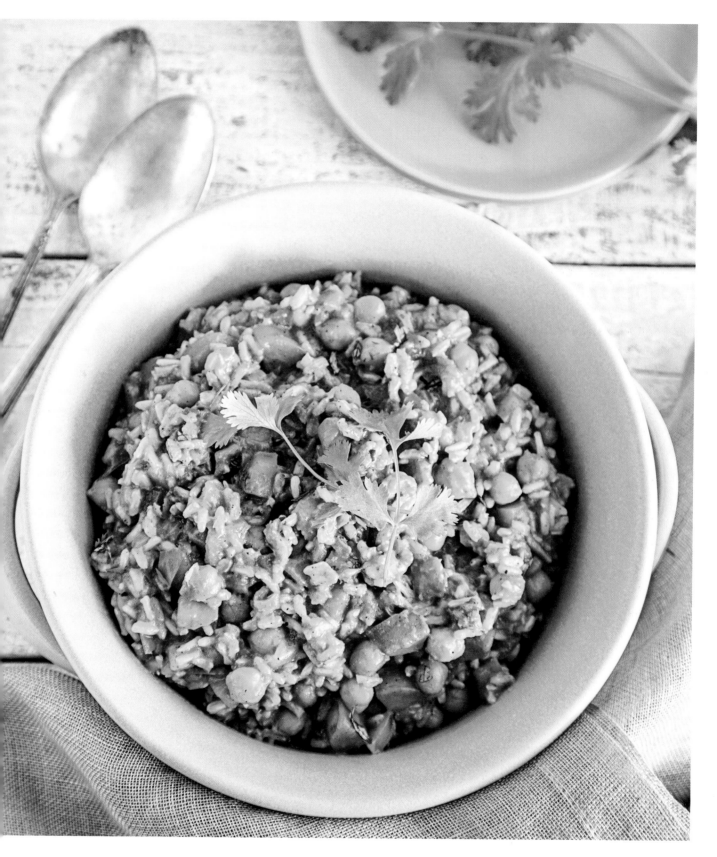

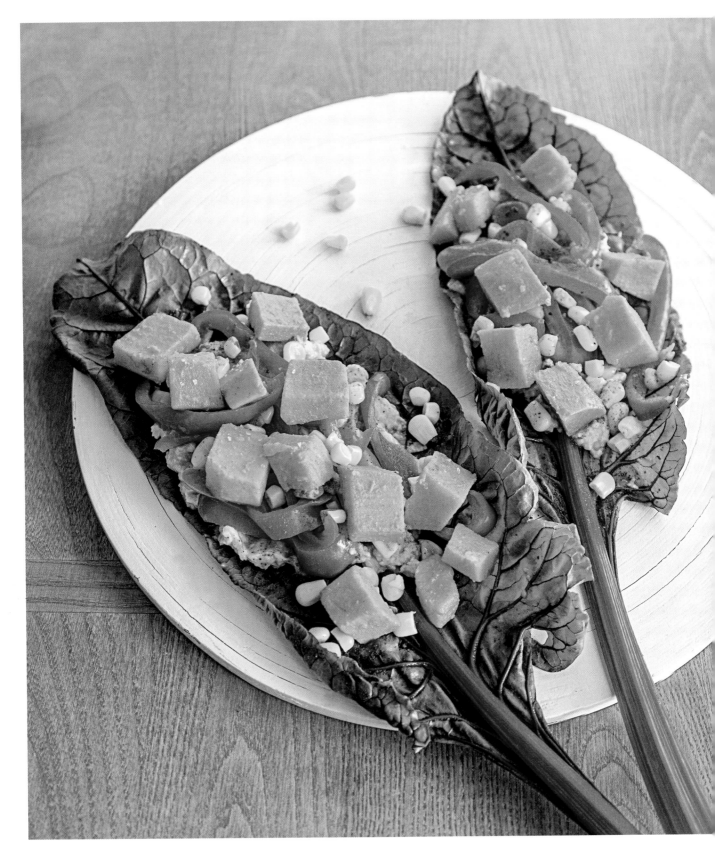

SWISS CHARD SWEET POTATO WRAPS

Chard is excellent for creating wraps, rolls and tacos. It tastes great raw or cooked, and paired with the right ingredients, this leafy green makes for a delicious and satisfying meal. For the filling, we prepared a simple avocado mash and paired it with a paprika-spiced sweet potato stuffing. Paprika is a great way to add color and flavor to your recipes. One tablespoon (7 g) contains over 70 percent of your vitamin A needs, and it also comes packed with lutein and zeaxanthin, two carotenoids that have been shown to have protective effects against eye disease.

Gluten-free / Vegan / 30 minutes or less

Serves: 1 / **Calories:** 440 / **Carbohydrates:** 59 g / **Protein:** 8 g / **Fat:** 21 g

- 1 cup (133 g) cubed sweet potato
- 2 tsp (10 ml) olive oil
- ½ red bell pepper, sliced into strips
- ½ cup cooked corn
- 1 tsp paprika
- ½ avocado
- ½ small onion, chopped
- Juice of ½ lime
- Salt and cayenne pepper to taste
- 2 large Swiss chard leaves

Boil the sweet potato cubes in a pot of water with the lid on for 15 minutes, until tender. Drain the water and set aside. Heat the olive oil in a pan over medium heat and add the red pepper slices, corn and cooked sweet potato. Season with the paprika and sauté for 4 to 5 minutes. Allow the mixture to cool.

In a bowl, combine the avocado, onion and lime juice. Using a fork or a pestle, mash the ingredients together until it resembles guacamole. Add salt and cayenne to taste and set aside.

To assemble the wraps, cut the tough stems from the chard at the point where it meets the leaf; this will make it easier to roll up. Scoop half the avocado spread onto the center of the bottom side of each leaf. Then add half of the sweet potato sauté to each leaf. Either wrap the leaves up like burritos or eat them like tortillas. Enjoy!

SIMPLE SPINACH POMEGRANATE FETA SALAD

The name of this salad pretty much tells you everything you need to know, but we'll go ahead and lay out all of the details anyway. Pomegranates are one of our absolute favorite fruits because they are sweet and add a burst of juiciness in each bite. And who would have thought that pom pom seeds (as we like to call 'em) are just as nutritious as they are delicious? They're a great source of antioxidants, which will help reboot your body by protecting your cells from free-radical damage. The spinach in this recipe will provide your daily dose of vitamin A (168 percent daily value) and vitamin C (42 percent), while the quinoa will help meet your complex carbohydrate and protein quotas.

Gluten-free / 30 minutes or less

Serves: 1 / **Calories:** 610 / **Carbohydrates:** 63 g / **Protein:** 17 g / **Fat:** 35 g

- ¾ cup (180 ml) water
- ¼ cup (43 g) uncooked quinoa
- Salt to taste

SALAD
- 3 cups (90 g) raw spinach
- ½ cup (87 g) pomegranate seeds
- ¼ cup (61 g) feta cheese
- 2 tsp (4.5 g) chopped pecans

CITRUS DRESSING
- 1 clove garlic
- 1 tsp olive oil
- Juice of ½ lime
- Juice of 1 mandarin orange
- Salt and pepper to taste

In a small pot, bring the water to a boil over high heat, and then add the quinoa. Lower the heat to a simmer, cover with a lid and cook for 15 to 17 minutes. When the quinoa is soft and fluffy, add salt to taste and allow it to cool.

For the salad, add the spinach, cooked quinoa, pom pom seeds, feta and pecans to a large bowl. Mix the salad together.

For the dressing, blend the dressing ingredients in a blender or food processor until smooth. If you don't have a blender or food processor, chop the garlic first, then mix all the ingredients in a bowl. Pour the dressing over the salad and eat your heart out.

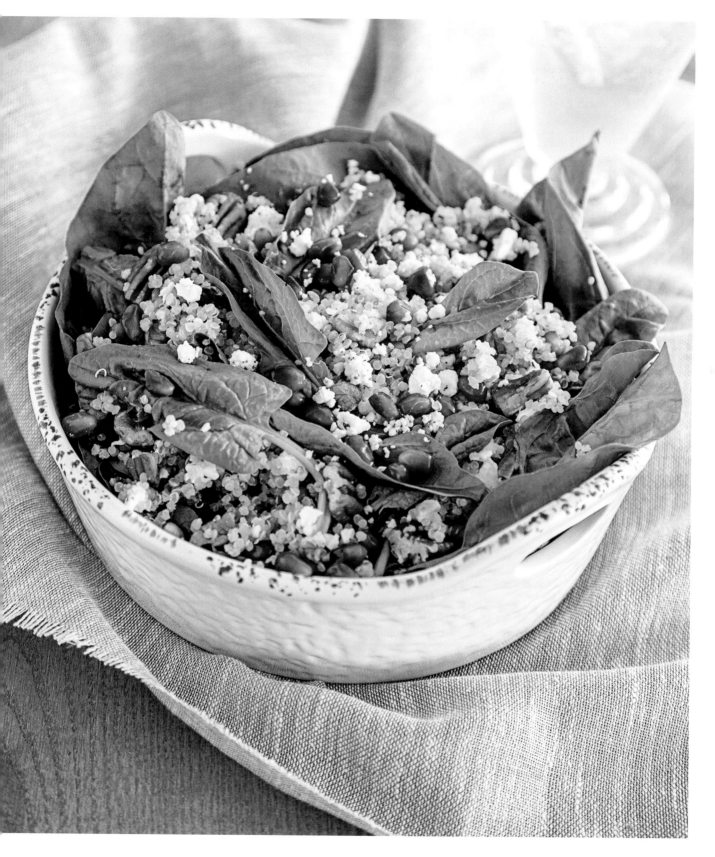

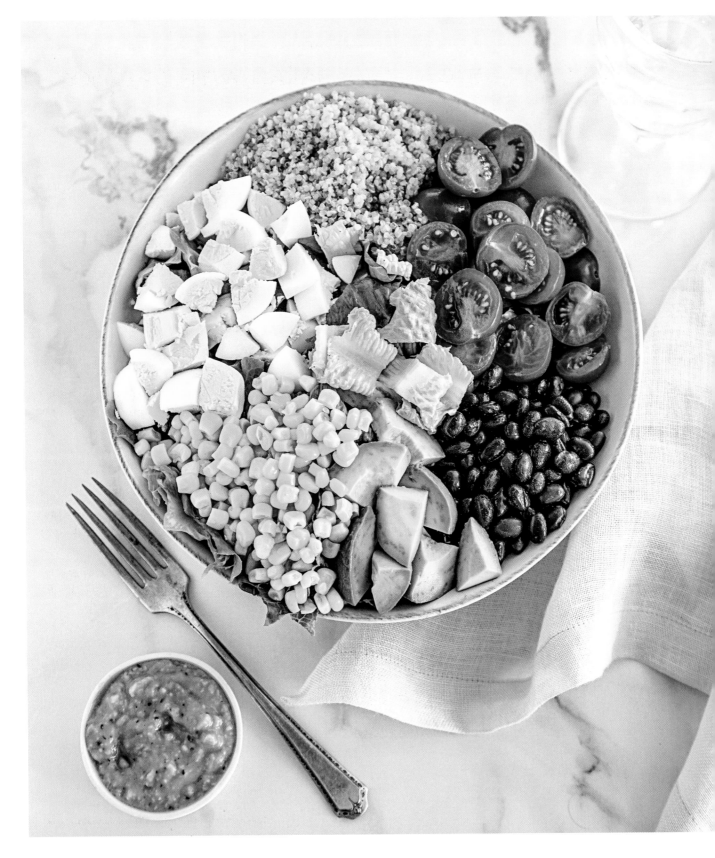

VEGETARIAN QUINOA COBB SALAD WITH CREAMY AVOCADO DRESSING

Wendy and I always see Cobb salads on hotel menus, but we figured they were off limits because there was meat involved. That was, until, we made our own. This Cobb salad is easy, delicious, nutritious and filling. You'll get nearly 3 cups (680 g) of veggies with this recipe alone, meeting almost 25 grams of your fiber needs for the day (fiber = beans, quinoa, lettuce + corn). Why do we love fiber so much? There are a million reasons. (Okay, maybe not a million, but definitely five.) One of the most important is that fiber helps strengthen the colon as it moves through your digestive tract. It also helps lower cholesterol, helps you feel full and prevents certain types of cancers. Now that we've gotten the health talk out of the way, let's get started with this tasty recipe.

Gluten-free / 30 minutes or less

Serves: 1 / **Calories:** 579 / **Carbohydrates:** 68 g / **Protein:** 28 g / **Fat:** 24 g

- ¾ cup (180 ml) water
- ¼ cup (45 g) uncooked quinoa
- Salt to taste

SALAD

- 2 cups (94 g) chopped romaine lettuce
- 10 cherry tomatoes
- 2 hard-boiled eggs
- ¼ avocado
- ⅓ cup (48 g) raw corn
- ½ cup (93 g) cooked black beans

DRESSING

- ¼ avocado
- Juice from ½ lemon
- 2 tsp (10 ml) rice vinegar
- 1 tsp water
- 1 clove garlic
- Salt and pepper to taste

In a small pot, bring the water to a boil over high heat, and then add the quinoa. Lower the heat to a simmer, cover with a lid and cook for 15–17 minutes. When the quinoa is soft and fluffy, add salt to taste and allow it to cool.

The secret to a successful Cobb salad is finely chopping everything so you can enjoy it in perfect little bites. Start by finely chopping the lettuce, tomatoes, eggs and avocado.

Add the chopped lettuce, tomatoes, eggs, avocado, corn, black beans and quinoa to a large bowl. For this salad, it's more fun if you add each ingredient into it's own section, rather than mixing everything together.

To make the dressing, blend the avocado, lemon juice, vinegar, water and garlic in a food processor or blender until well mixed. Add salt and pepper to taste. Drizzle the salad with the creamy dressing and enjoy.

WHOLE-WHEAT PEARL COUSCOUS SALAD

Don't let the simplicity of this recipe fool you. It may have minimal ingredients but it delivers maximum flavor. The trick here is jazzing up the couscous by cooking it in vegetable broth. We love pearl couscous (also known as Israeli couscous) specifically because it's flat out more fun (for us) than its traditional couscous counterpart, which is made up of smaller granules. Pearl couscous offers an alternative to the popular brown rice and quinoa for many dishes. It's also really easy to cook—simply add it to boiling water and cook for about 10 minutes and it's ready to go.

30 minutes or less

Serves: 1 / **Calories:** 505 / **Carbohydrates:** 78 g / **Protein:** 20 g / **Fat:** 11 g

- 1 cup (237 ml) water
- 1 cup (237 ml) vegetable broth
- ½ cup (86 g) uncooked whole-wheat pearl couscous
- ¼ cucumber
- ¼ cup (14 g) sliced sun-dried tomatoes
- ⅓ cup (81 g) feta cheese
- Salt and pepper to taste

Bring the water and veggie broth to a boil in a small saucepan, add the couscous, reduce to a simmer and cook for about 10 minutes, or until the water is absorbed. Transfer to a bowl.

While the couscous cooks, chop the cucumber into ½-inch (1.3-cm) cubes.

Add the cucumber, sun-dried tomatoes and feta cheese to the cooked couscous. As you mix the ingredients, the cheese will start to melt a bit and the result will give a thick and somewhat creamy consistency to the salad. Season with salt and pepper to taste.

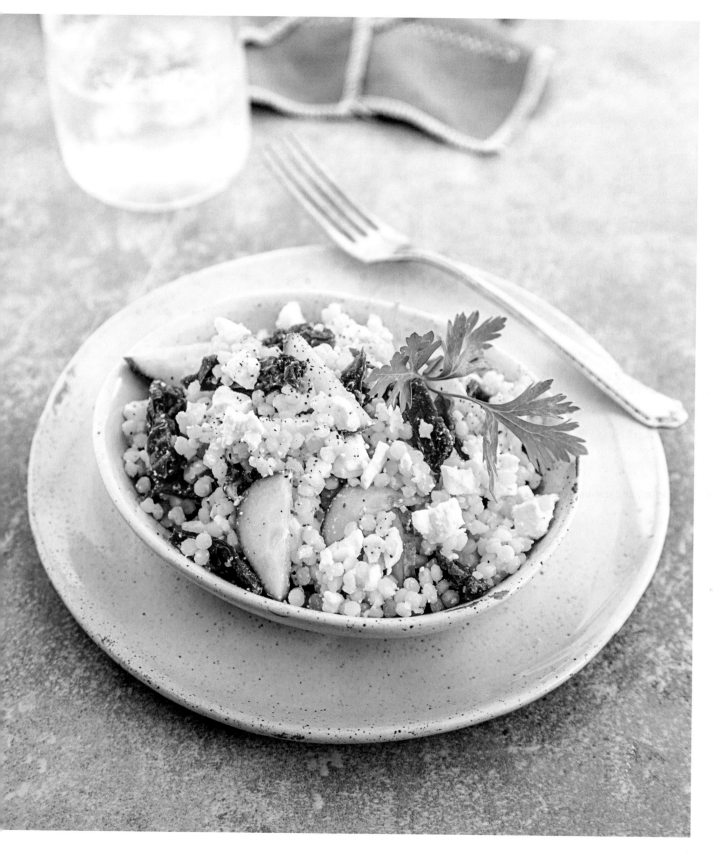

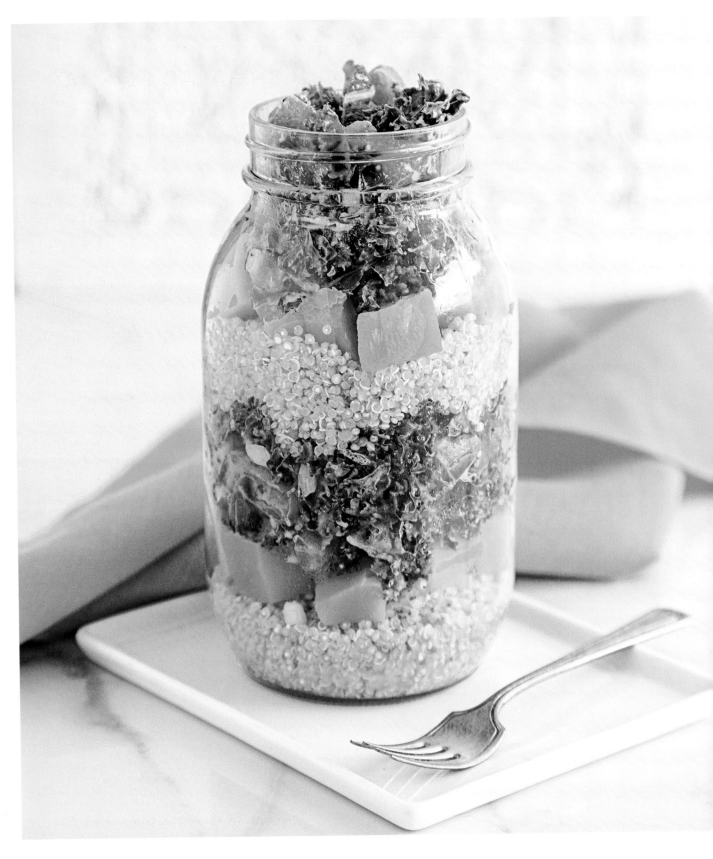

CREAMY KALE BUTTERNUT SQUASH SALAD IN A JAR

This creamy salad is perfection bottled up in a jar. It's made with nourishing ingredients that shine even brighter when enjoyed together. The butternut squash provides a rich source of vitamins A and C. We're also getting protein and complex carbohydrates thanks to the hummus and quinoa. Salads don't get any better than this!

Gluten-free / Vegan / 30 minutes or less

Serves: 1 / **Calories:** 462 / **Carbohydrates:** 55 g / **Protein:** 16 g / **Fat:** 15 g

- ¾ cup (177 ml) water
- ¼ cup (42 g) uncooked quinoa
- Salt and cayenne pepper to taste
- ¾ cup (105 g) peeled and chopped butternut squash
- 2 cups (32 g) chopped kale
- ¼ cup (61 g) hummus
- 1 small tomato, cubed
- ¼ small onion, chopped
- 1 tsp olive oil

Bring the water to a boil in a small pot, add the quinoa, cover with the lid, lower the heat and cook for 15 to 17 minutes, until the quinoa is soft and fluffy. Add salt to taste and allow it to cool.

Meanwhile, boil the butternut squash chunks in a pot of water with the lid on for 20 minutes. Once you can easily stick a fork through the squash, remove it from the heat, drain the water and allow the squash to cool.

In a bowl, combine the kale, hummus, tomato, onion and olive oil. Using your hands, massage all of the ingredients together. Add salt and cayenne pepper to taste.

Now assemble your salad jar. Add some quinoa to the bottom of the jar, then some of the butternut squash and then some of the kale mixture. Repeat the layers until all of the ingredients have filled your jar. Let the flavors marinate in the refrigerator for at least an hour before enjoying. You can also assemble this the night before, store it in the refrigerator and then pack it up for lunch the next day! Enjoy your salad cold or reheat it for 1 minute if you prefer it warm.

ROASTED BRUSSELS SPROUTS GOAT CHEESE SALAD

This savory roasted Brussels sprouts salad is both filling and flavorful. The almighty sweet potato adds a subtle sweetness to the dish, and comes packed with fiber, vitamins A and C and trace mineral manganese. Complementing the sweet potato with Brussels sprouts makes this dish that much more nutritive. These two ingredients alone cover one third of your daily fiber needs! Add the creamy goat cheese and crunchy walnuts and you've got yourself a winner.

Gluten-free (if using gluten-free soy sauce)

Serves: 1 / **Calories:** 421 / **Carbohydrates:** 46 g / **Protein:** 15 g / **Fat:** 21 g

- 1 medium sweet potato, cut in half
- 2 cups (176 g) halved Brussels sprouts
- 1 tsp soy sauce
- 2 tsp (10 ml) olive oil
- 1 tbsp (7 g) chopped walnuts
- 1 oz (28 g) goat cheese
- 1 tbsp (10 ml) balsamic vinegar
- Salt and cayenne pepper to taste

Preheat the oven to 400°F (204°C). Line a baking sheet with aluminum foil.

Bring a pot of water to a boil over high heat. Add the sweet potato, then lower the heat and cook for 20 minutes. Remove the sweet potato from the pot and let it cool. When the sweet potato is cool, chop it into 1-inch (1.3-cm) cubes and place the cubes on the aluminum foil. Add the Brussels sprouts to the foil. Drizzle the sweet potatoes and Brussels sprouts with the soy sauce and olive oil, wrap them in the foil and pop them into the oven for 20 minutes. Remove them from the oven and let cool.

Place the roasted sweet potatoes and Brussels sprouts in a bowl. Add the walnuts and goat cheese and drizzle with the balsamic vinegar. Finish off with salt and cayenne pepper to taste. You can enjoy this salad warm or cold!

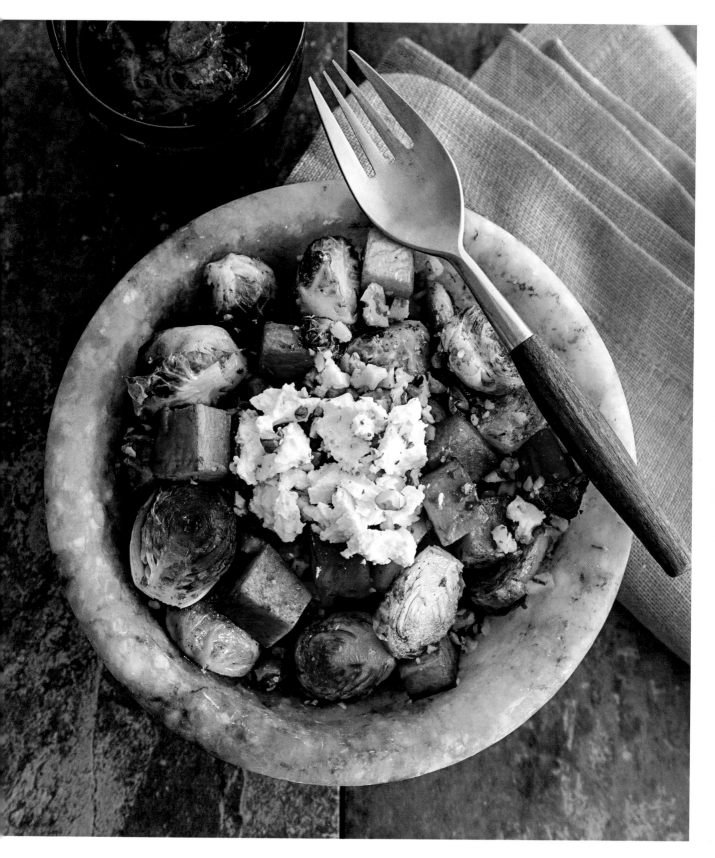

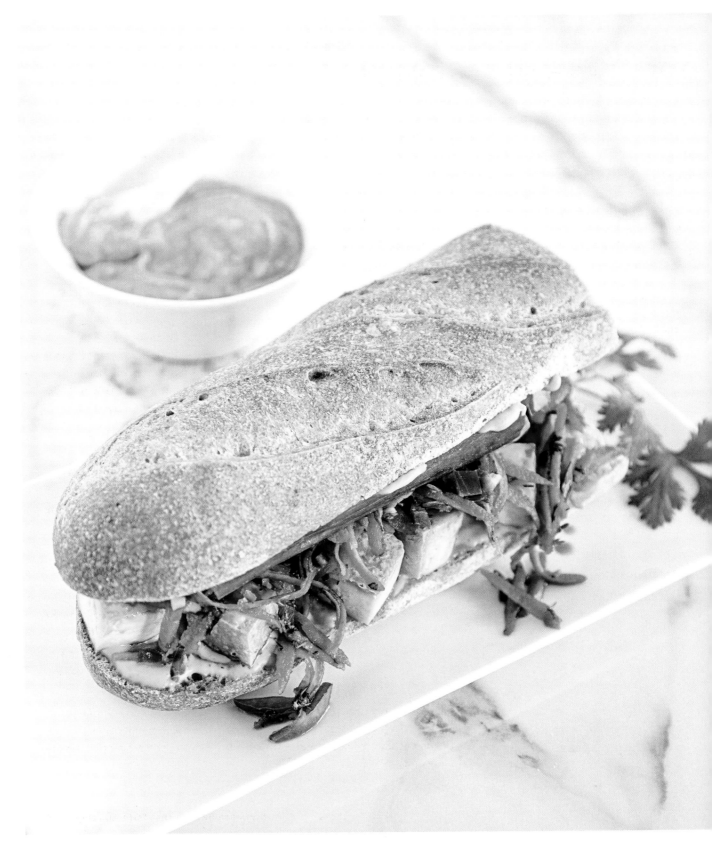

TOFU BANH MI SANDWICH

The banh mi is one of our absolute favorite sandwiches. Whenever we go to a Vietnamese restaurant and see a (vegetarian) banh mi on the menu, you bet we're ordering it. Maybe it's the French bread. Or the spicy mayo. Or the tiny burst of sweetness you get when you bite into the carrots and onions. Whatever it is, the banh mi makes our taste buds rejoice. In this recipe, we make our own two-ingredient spiced mayo that we think you'll love. We also focus on the vegetables to make sure you get a dose of fiber with each bite, which will help strengthen your colon and leave you feeling full and satisfied after your meal.

Serves: 1 / **Calories:** 565 / **Carbohydrates:** 59 g / **Protein:** 27 g / **Fat:** 26 g

- ½ (16-oz [454-g]) package extra-firm tofu or ½ cup (126 g) leftover cooked crispy tofu
- 4 tsp (20 g) light mayonnaise
- ½ tsp Sriracha
- ¼ carrot
- ¼ red onion
- 1 clove garlic, minced
- 1 small handful cilantro
- 2 tsp (10 ml) rice vinegar
- 1 tsp brown sugar
- 1 tsp soy sauce
- 1 whole-wheat French baguette
- ⅓ cucumber, sliced lengthwise
- ½ jalapeño pepper

If you don't have any leftover crispy tofu from previous recipes, you can make it from scratch here. Remove the tofu from the package and cut it in half. Submerge the remaining tofu in water in an airtight container. Store in the refrigerator and use for another recipe within 3 to 5 days. Wrap the half of the tofu you will be using for this recipe in a clean towel. Place in a glass pan, then put something heavy on top. The idea is to press all of the water out of the tofu for up to 4 hours. When the tofu is drained, cut it into small cubes (about ½ x ½-inch [1.3 x 1.3-cm]).

Preheat the oven to 375°F (190°C). Oil a baking sheet.

Spread the cubed tofu on the prepared baking sheet and bake for 30 minutes, flipping the tofu with a spatula halfway through. Remove from the oven and increase the heat to 400°F (204°C). Store any cooked tofu that you don't use in an airtight container in the refrigerator for up to 1 week.

To make the super easy Sriracha mayo, combine and stir the mayonnaise and Sriracha until you have a creamy pink mayo. Set aside.

Grate the carrot and thinly slice the onion. Mince the garlic and chop the cilantro. Place all of these ingredients in a bowl then add the vinegar, brown sugar and soy sauce. Massage the ingredients together with your hands, then set aside.

To toast the baguette, slice it lengthwise and place it directly on the rack in the 400°F (204°C) oven. Toast for 3 to 5 minutes. While the baguette is toasting, slice the cucumber lengthwise, and seed and chop the jalapeño into rounds.

Spread the mayo on both slices of the toasted baguette. Add a layer of tofu (you can reheat this if you choose) on one half of the baguette, then the carrot and onion mixture and the cucumber and jalapeño. Top with the remaining baguette half and enjoy!

SPICY OPEN-FACED AVOCADO SANDWICH

This is one of our favorite go-to quick recipes. Our motto is that delicious doesn't have to be complicated. In fact, the simplest recipes are usually the tastiest (not to mention healthiest). This recipe is packed with a balance of protein, fat and carbohydrates, so it will keep you full for hours. You'll also get a good amount of essential vitamins and minerals. For example, avocados are packed with vitamin E, copper, folate and pantothenic acid, and the cheese will give you a hefty dose of calcium, phosphorous and even a little bit of B_{12}. Make sure you purchase whole-wheat (or whole-grain) bread that contains about 5 grams of fiber or more per serving.

30 minutes or less

Serves: 1 / **Calories:** 512 / **Carbohydrates:** 53 g / **Protein:** 23 g / **Fat:** 26 g

- **2 slices 100% whole-wheat bread**
- **2 tsp (10 g) hummus**
- **⅓ avocado**
- **1 small Roma tomato**
- **2 slices pepper Jack cheese**
- **Crushed red pepper flakes and salt to taste**

Preheat the toaster or oven to 375°F (190°C). Toast the bread to your desired doneness. Remove the bread, but keep the toaster or oven on. Spread the hummus on each slice of toast.

Finely slice the avocado and divide the slices between your two pieces of toast. Do the same with the tomato—slice and divide. Finally, add a slice of cheese to each and then place in the oven for about 3 minutes, or until the cheese has melted. Top with a sprinkle of red pepper flakes and salt to taste.

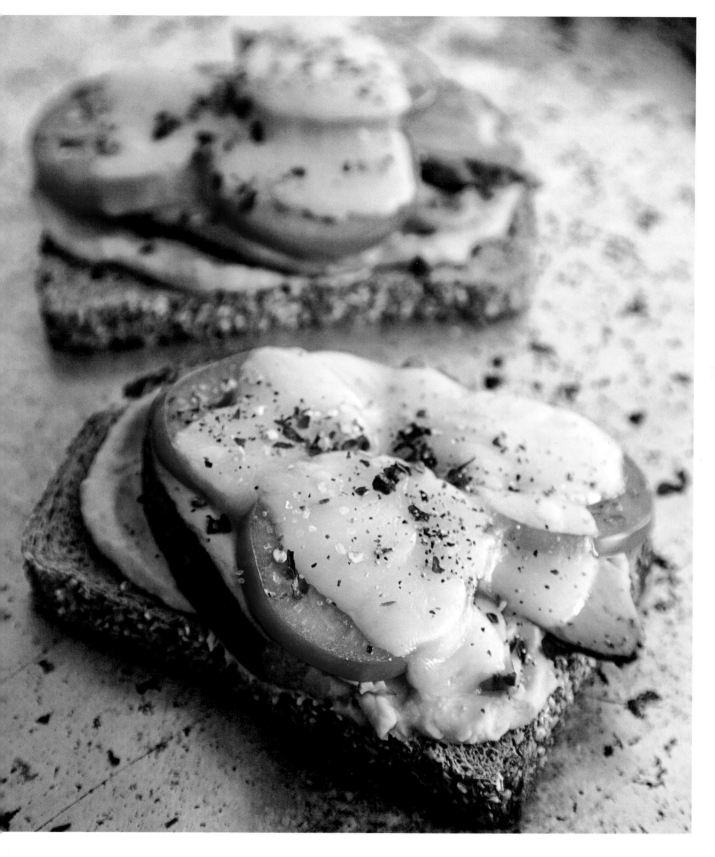

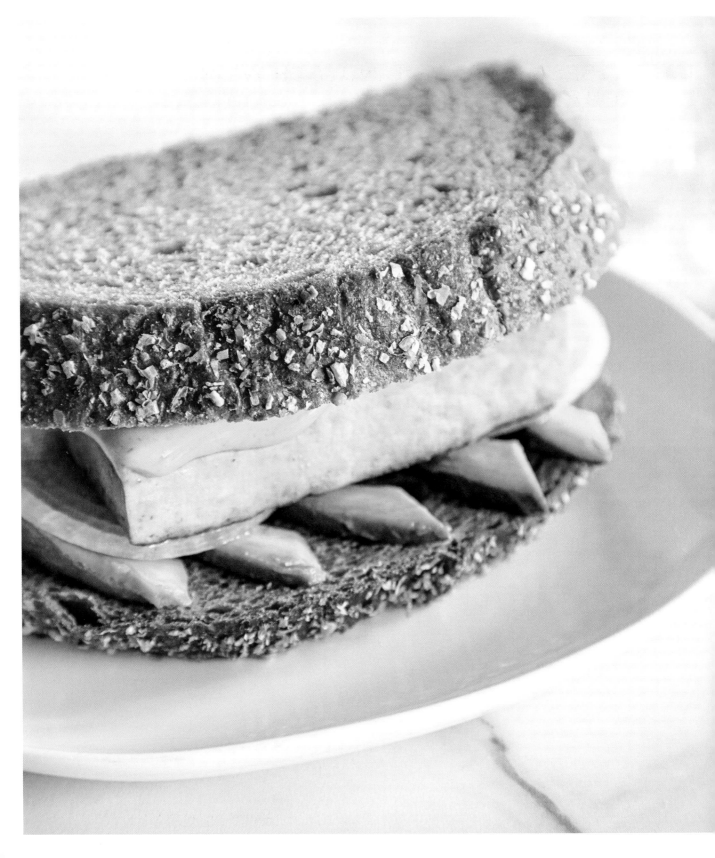

GARLIC SESAME TOFU SANDWICH WITH SRIRACHA MAYO

Tofu is often used as a sponge in recipes. It soaks up all of the wonderful flavors you cook it in, which in this case makes for a pretty remarkable sandwich. The simple marinade for soaking the tofu adds a nutty aroma and taste, plus a beautiful deep-brown color. Tofu is a great way to add protein, calcium and iron to your meals. Because of its versatility in the kitchen, it can be used in smoothies, desserts, stews and much more!

30 minutes or less

Serves: 1 / **Calories:** 372 / **Carbohydrates:** 34 g / **Protein:** 17 g / **Fat:** 21 g

- ⅛ block firm tofu
- 1 tsp sesame seed oil
- 1 tsp soy sauce
- ½ tsp rice vinegar
- ¼ tsp garlic powder
- 2 slices 100% whole-grain bread
- ¼ avocado, sliced
- 3 onion rounds
- ½ tsp light mayonnaise
- 1 tsp Sriracha

Place the tofu in a bowl and add the sesame seed oil, soy sauce, rice vinegar and garlic powder. Flip the tofu over so that both sides are coated well with the marinade. You can also use a spoon to help get the marinade onto the tofu. Allow the tofu to marinate for at least 15 minutes. Then place the tofu on a grill press and cook for 8 to 9 minutes, or until the tofu has a deep golden-brown color. If using the stove, cook the tofu in a pan over medium heat for 3 minutes on each side.

To arrange your sandwich, lay your 2 slices of bread on a plate and add the avocado, onion and cooked tofu on one slice. On the other slice, add the mayonnaise and Sriracha. Using a butter knife, spread these two ingredients together well. Place this slice on top of the layered tofu slice and enjoy!

GREEN GODDESS SANDWICH

The original green goddess dressing uses mayonnaise, sour cream and herbs to create a thick and rich spread. We created this vegan alternative, using the creaminess of hummus with the sweetness of fresh basil, to create a filling spread that seamlessly brings together all of the other ingredients. Hummus is a great way to boost the fiber, protein and heart-healthy fat content of your meals. Add it to salads, wraps, toast and even soups!

Vegan / 30 minutes or less

Serves: 1 / **Calories:** 410 / **Carbohydrates:** 58 g / **Protein:** 17 g / **Fat:** 13 g

- 3 tbsp (46 g) hummus
- 5 fresh basil leaves
- 1 scallion
- 2 slices 100% whole-grain bread
- ¼ cup (7.5 g) raw spinach
- ¼ avocado, sliced
- 3 yellow onion rounds
- Salt and black pepper to taste

Add the hummus, fresh basil and scallion to a food processor. Blend until the basil and scallion have been broken down, and you have a creamy, green spread. Place the bread on a plate. Using a butter knife, apply the spread evenly on each slice of bread. On one of the slices, add the spinach, avocado and onion. Sprinkle with salt and pepper to taste and top with the other slice of bread. Enjoy!

MEDITERRANEAN BUDDHA BOWL WITH ROASTED CHICKPEAS

If there is one bowl that completely revolutionized the way we lunch in 2016, it is the Buddha bowl. A Buddha bowl is quite simple at its core. All you do is throw a bunch of complementary ingredients in a bowl and enjoy. Of course, there are many fancy variations to this dish (a quick Pinterest search will reveal more than a thousand combinations), but we wanted to make things super easy for you, the busy home chef. The key here is using only the freshest ingredients, so the flavors speak for themselves without much manipulation (cooking) from the chef (you).

Vegan

Serves: 1 / **Calories:** 613 / **Carbohydrates:** 77 g / **Protein:** 19 g / **Fat:** 26 g

- ¼ **red bell pepper**
- ¼ **yellow bell pepper**
- 1 tsp **olive oil, divided**
- ½ tsp **dried oregano**
- **Salt and pepper to taste**
- ½ cup (82 g) **cooked chickpeas**
- 1 tsp **smoked paprika**
- **A pinch of cayenne pepper**
- ½ tsp **chopped mint**
- ¼ **cucumber, chopped**
- 2½ tbsp (40 ml) **lemon juice, divided**
- ⅓ cup (44 g) **pitted black olives**
- 6 **cherry tomatoes, chopped**
- ½ cup (10 g) **chopped arugula**
- ½ cup (93 g) **cooked quinoa**
- ¼ cup (62 g) **hummus**
- ½ **100% whole-wheat pita**

Preheat the oven to 425°F (218°C). Line an 18 x 13-inch (46 x 33-cm) baking sheet with parchment paper. Get out a large bowl with a good amount of surface area so that all of the Buddha bowl ingredients will fit and look pretty.

Chop the red and yellow peppers and add to a mixing bowl. Add ½ teaspoon of the olive oil, the dried oregano and a pinch of salt and stir or toss to coat the peppers. Spread the peppers on the prepared baking sheet, covering about half of the sheet.

Rinse and drain the chickpeas, then pat them dry with a towel as much as possible (less water = more crunchy). Add the chickpeas to the same mixing bowl used for the peppers and add the remaining ½ teaspoon olive oil, the paprika and cayenne pepper. Stir or toss to coat the chickpeas then add them to the other half of the baking sheet. Roast the peppers and chickpeas for 30 to 35 minutes, flipping the chickpeas and peppers every 10 minutes or so.

While the peppers and chickpeas are roasting, combine the mint, cucumber, a sprinkle of salt and 1 tablespoon (16 ml) of the lemon juice in a small bowl and stir to blend. Add the cucumber mix to one corner of your Buddha bowl. Then add the olives, tomatoes and arugula to another corner. Drizzle the remaining 1½ tablespoons (24 ml) lemon juice over the chopped tomatoes and arugula for a tangy twist. Finally, add the roasted chickpeas and peppers and then the cooked quinoa to the remaining two corners, with a tiny bit of salt and pepper to flavor the quinoa to taste. Add the hummus to the middle of the bowl. Toast the pita bread, then slice into triangles to serve with your Buddha bowl. Dig in!

*See photo on page 26.

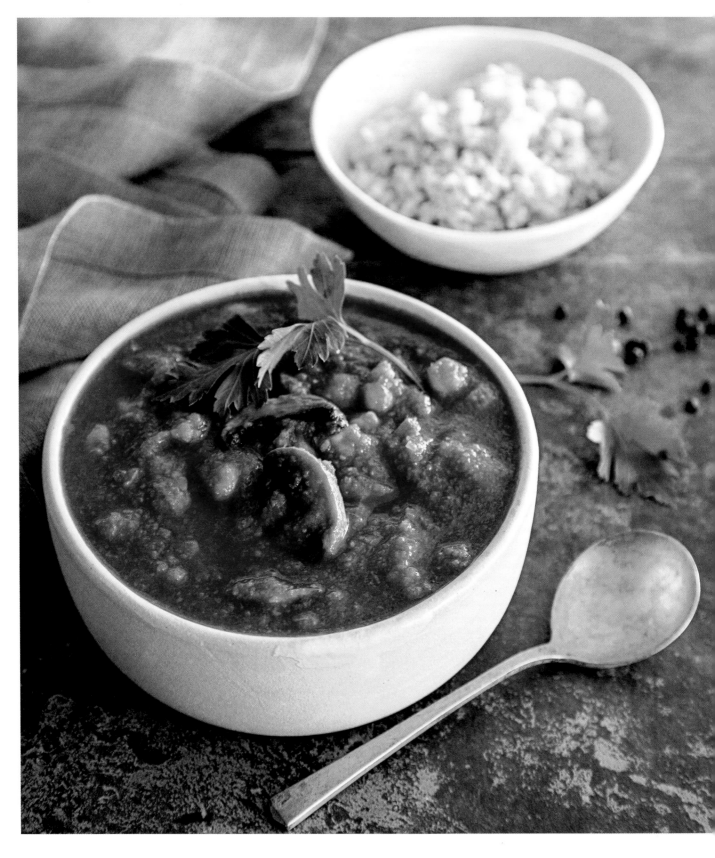

SAVORY MUSHROOM CARROT STEW

This savory stew has a pinch of sweetness from the carrots and all the savory goodness of the onions and peppers. The thick consistency of the stew results from first cooking the carrots, and then blending them into a purée. This stew is paired with fiber-rich bulgur, a whole grain that cooks quickly and goes well with so many great dishes!

Vegan / 30 minutes or less

Serves: 2

Per Serving / Calories: 511 / **Carbohydrates:** 82 g / **Protein:** 18 g / **Fat:** 12 g

- 6 medium carrots, peeled
- 4 tsp (20 ml) olive oil
- 2 tbsp (33 g) tomato paste
- ½ medium onion, chopped
- 1 red bell pepper, seeded and chopped
- 2 cups (144 g) sliced button mushrooms
- 1 cup (164 g) cooked chickpeas
- 2 cups (473 ml) water
- Salt and cayenne pepper to taste
- 1 cup (182 g) cooked cracked bulgur

Bring a pot of water to a boil over high heat. Chop the carrots into 2 or 3 smaller pieces, add to the boiling water, lower the heat to medium-low, and cook for 10 to 15 minutes, or until tender. Drain the carrots, reserving ¼ cup (60 ml) of the cooking water. Allow the carrots to cool and add them to a food processor with the reserved cooking water. Blend into a purée and then set aside.

Heat the olive oil in a pot over medium heat, then add the tomato paste, onion and bell pepper. Sauté for 2 to 3 minutes, then add the mushrooms and chickpeas, along with the carrot purée and 2 cups (473 ml) of water. Mix everything together with a large spoon and cover with a lid. Cook for 10 minutes over medium-low heat. Season with salt and pepper to taste and enjoy with 1 serving (½ cup [91 g]) of the cooked bulgur.

LENTIL SLOPPY JOES

Who else had sloppy joes on the school lunch menu when growing up? One thing's for sure, our vegan sloppy joes are a whole lot better. We love this lentil variation on a traditional dish because they aren't as "sloppy" as traditional sloppy joes, making them easier to eat, and they are jam-packed with nutrition, especially protein and fiber. In fact, just 1 cup (192 g) of lentils has a whopping 18 grams of protein and 16 grams of fiber. Not to mention, these taste absolutely delicious and are the perfect filling, flavorful meal for your weekday lunch.

Vegan / 30 minutes or less

Serves: 2
Per Serving / Calories: 443 / **Carbohydrates:** 67 g / **Protein:** 26 g / **Fat:** 7 g

- 1½ cups (288 g) dried lentils
- 2 tsp (10 ml) olive oil
- ½ cup (120 g) canned diced tomatoes
- ½ cup (132 g) tomato paste
- 2 cloves garlic, chopped
- ⅓ jalapeño, seeded and chopped
- 4 tsp (20 ml) apple cider vinegar
- 1 tsp paprika
- 2 tsp (5 g) chili powder
- 1 tsp ground cumin
- 1 tsp cooking wine
- Salt to taste
- 2 firm 100% whole-wheat hamburger buns or rolls

Bring a pot of water to a boil over high heat, add the lentils, then reduce the heat to medium-low and simmer for about 20 minutes, or until tender. Drain and let cool.

Heat the olive oil in a skillet over medium heat. Tip: If you want to make sure the oil is heated before adding food, place your hand an inch or two (2.5 to 5 cm) above the pan. If it feels warm, it's ready to go. If not, leave it be for another minute or so. Toss in the diced tomatoes and tomato paste, stir and cook for 3 minutes. Add the chopped garlic and jalapeño, then cook for another 2 minutes. Add the cooked lentils, vinegar, paprika, chili powder, ground cumin and cooking wine. Lower the heat and simmer for 3 to 5 minutes, stirring frequently. If it gets dry, add a teaspoon of water as needed. Season with salt to taste.

Open the hamburger buns and toast each side in the toaster or oven. Stuff with the lentils and enjoy!

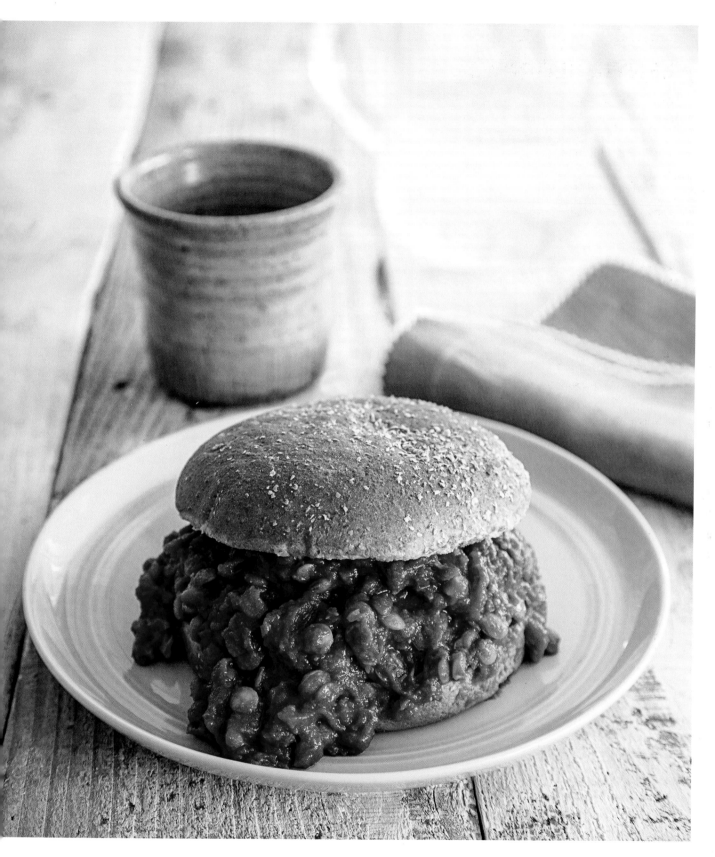

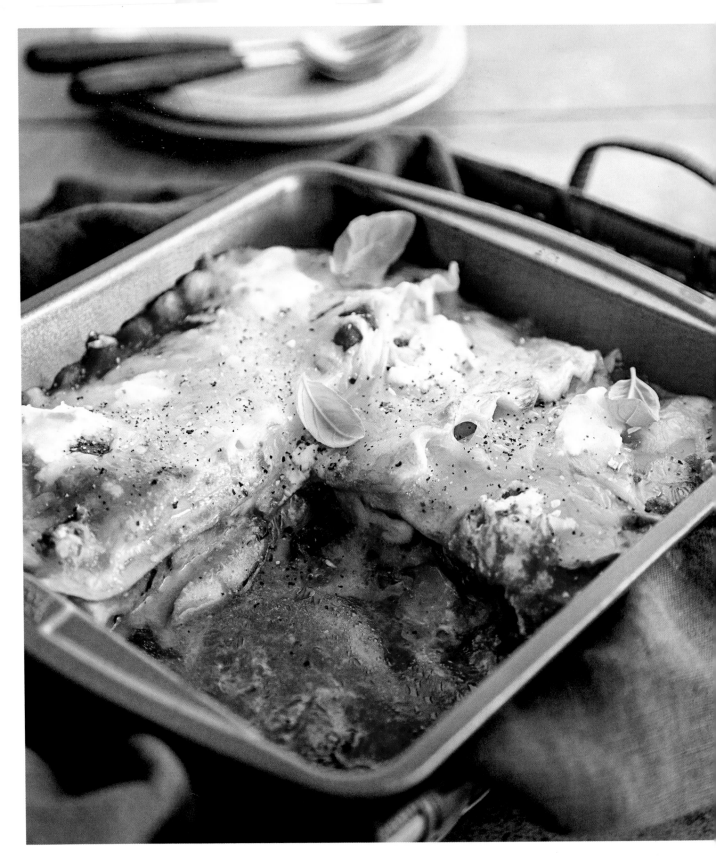

VEGETABLE LAYERED LASAGNA

This hearty vegetable lasagna is a lighter alternative to the traditional lasagna. We used both pasta and zucchini to create the layers and made a savory Swiss chard and mushroom sauté for the filling. Swiss chard is one of those vegetables that doesn't get enough shine. It can be incorporated into dishes in so many ways and provides a hefty dose of vitamins A, C and K. Throw the leaves (and stems!) into stews, soups, sautés, smoothies and more!

Serves: 2

Per Serving / **Calories:** 463 / **Carbohydrates:** 57 g / **Protein:** 24 g / **Fat:** 17 g

- 1 tbsp (15 ml) olive oil
- ½ medium onion, chopped
- 2 cups (60 g) finely chopped Swiss chard
- 2 cups (144 g) sliced button mushrooms
- 2 medium zucchini
- 6 lasagna noodles
- 1 cup (245 g) tomato sauce
- ½ cup (124 g) light ricotta cheese
- ½ cup (57 g) shredded mozzarella cheese
- Salt and black pepper to taste

Preheat the oven to 400°F (204°C).

Heat the olive oil in a skillet over medium heat and add the chopped onion. Sauté for 1 to 2 minutes, and then add the chard and mushrooms. Sauté for 4 to 5 minutes, and then set aside.

Trim the ends, then slice each zucchini lengthwise into four slices, and set aside.

Cook the noodles as per package instructions, making sure the cooked noodles are pliable but still firm. You can skip this step by using no-cook lasagna noodles.

Coat an 8 x 8-inch (20.5 x 20.5-cm) baking dish with a thin layer of tomato sauce, and top with three closely aligned, but not overlapping, lasagna noodles. If the noodles don't fit the baking dish you're using, you can cut them so they match the pan size. Add another thin layer of the tomato sauce, half the vegetable sauté, one-third of the ricotta cheese and one-third of the mozzarella cheese onto the noodles. Then add the four zucchini slices, some tomato sauce, the remaining half of the vegetable sauté, and one third of each of the cheeses. Cover with the remaining three lasagna noodles and the remaining tomato sauce, ricotta and mozzarella.

Bake for 25 minutes, or until bubbling around the edges and golden on top. Let cool. Season with salt and black pepper to taste and enjoy!

SIMPLE FRIED EGG AND QUINOA AVOCADO POWER BOWL

This simple power bowl is easy to make and super satisfying to the tummy. It's one of our go-to recipes when there's "nothing" to eat in the kitchen. But don't let the simplicity fool you. This basic recipe offers the maximum nutritional benefit. For example, did you know that eggs are a perfect protein because they contain all of the essential amino acids in the desired ratios? Eggs are also one of the highest-content food sources of leucine, an essential amino acid that helps trigger muscle protein synthesis. We also add a healthy dose of avocado because pairing a fat with carotenoid-rich foods, like the tomatoes in this recipe, will help with the absorption of this phytonutrient. Nutrition aside, give this easy lunch idea a try!

Gluten-free / 30 minutes or less

Serves: 1 / **Calories:** 414 / **Carbohydrates:** 46 g / **Protein:** 15 g / **Fat:** 19 g

- 1 cup (240 ml) water
- ⅓ cup (60 g) uncooked quinoa
- Salt to taste
- ⅓ tomato
- ½ clove garlic
- ½ shallot
- ⅛ jalapeño, seeded
- Juice of ⅛ lemon
- ½ tsp olive oil
- ¼ tsp fresh thyme
- ½ tsp dried oregano
- ⅛ avocado
- 1 tsp vegetable oil
- 1 egg

In a small pot, bring the water to a boil over high heat, and then add the quinoa. Lower the heat to a simmer, cover with a lid and cook for 15 to 17 minutes. When the quinoa is soft and fluffy, add salt to taste and allow it to cool.

To make the salsa, finely chop the tomato, garlic, shallot and jalapeño, then add to a bowl along with the lemon juice. Stir to combine.

In a serving bowl, mix the cooked quinoa with the olive oil, thyme and oregano. Slice the avocado and lay the slices over one corner of the quinoa. Set aside.

Heat the vegetable oil in a pan over medium-high heat. Crack the egg into the pan and cook for 3 to 5 minutes, or until the bottom is slightly crispy and the yolk starts to firm up. Remove the egg and place on top of your quinoa bowl. Sprinkle with salt. Spoon the salsa over the top. Time to eat!

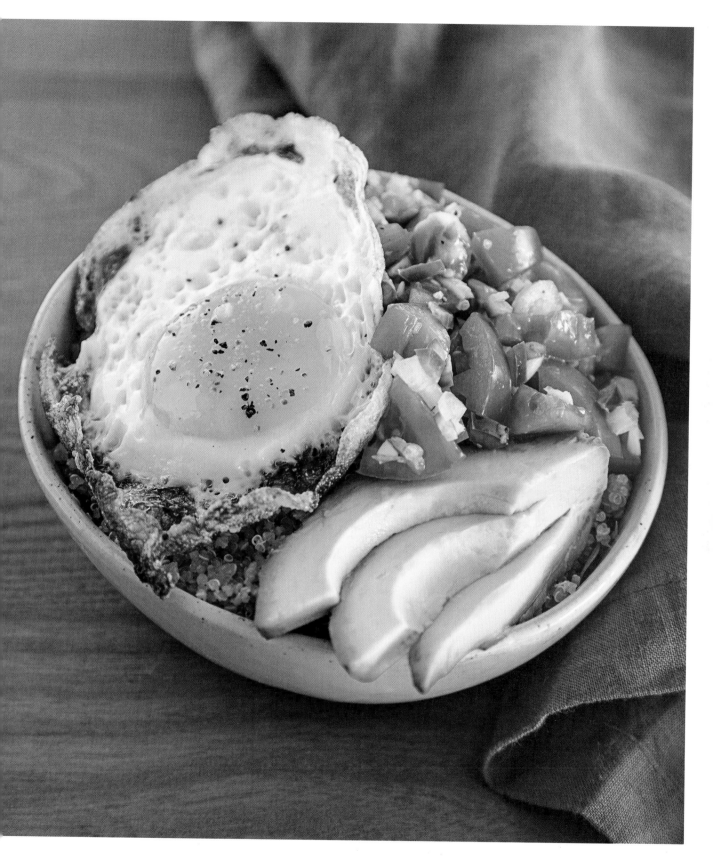

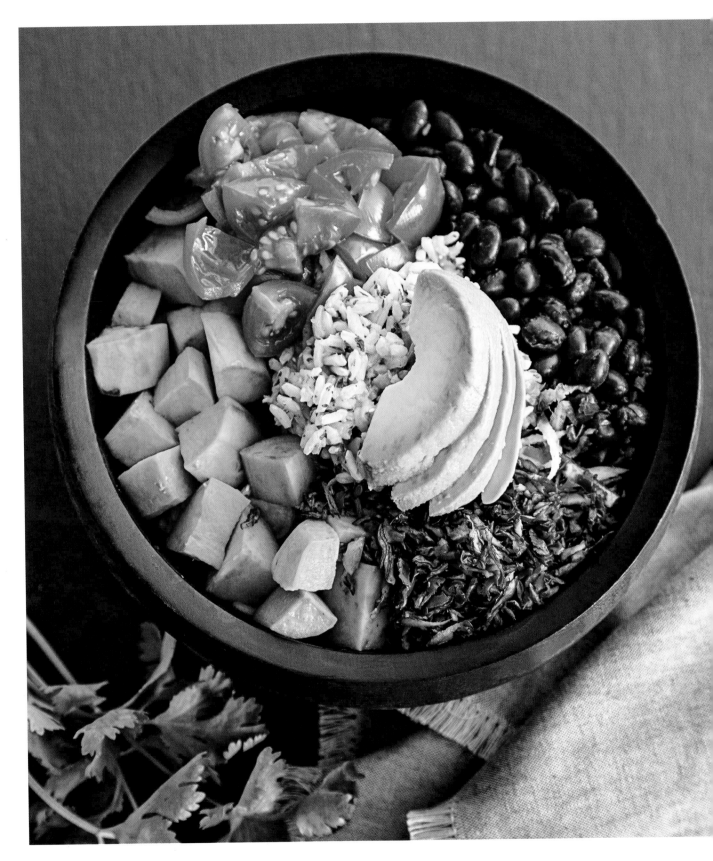

SWEET POTATO BURRITO BOWL WITH GREEN RICE

What beats going out to buy a burrito bowl? Making one yourself! This tasty sweet potato burrito bowl starts with throwing really fresh, flavorful ingredients together . . . and what happens next is magic. Aside from being absolutely delicious, this burrito bowl covers more than 70 percent of your fiber needs for an entire day! It's packed with heart-healthy fats to keep you satiated, too.

Gluten-free / Vegan

Serves: 1 / **Calories:** 462 / **Carbohydrates:** 78 g / **Protein:** 14 g / **Fat:** 13 g

- ½ cup (67 g) cubed sweet potato
- 1 tsp olive oil
- 1 tsp maple syrup
- 2 sprigs fresh thyme
- 1 cup plus 2 tbsp (266 ml) water, divided
- ¼ cup (48 g) raw brown rice
- ½ cup (25 g) fresh cilantro
- ½ jalapeño, seeded and chopped
- ¼ small onion, chopped
- Salt to taste
- ½ cup (93 g) cooked black beans
- ¼ cup (45 g) cubed tomato
- ¼ cup (18 g) grated red cabbage
- ¼ avocado, sliced
- Juice of ½ lime

Preheat the oven to 400°F (204°C). Line a baking sheet with aluminum foil.

Place the sweet potato cubes on the foil, drizzle with the olive oil and maple syrup, tuck in the thyme sprigs and fold up the foil. Bake for 25 minutes, or until the sweet potatoes are tender.

Bring 1 cup (237 ml) of the water to a boil in a small pot, add the brown rice, cover with a lid, reduce the heat to low, and cook for 20 to 25 minutes, or until the rice is tender. Set aside.

While the sweet potato is baking and the rice is cooking, add the cilantro, jalapeño, onion and remaining 2 tablespoons (30 ml) water to a blender. Pulse a few times until all of the ingredients are blended. Add the green sauce to the finished pot of rice and mix it in well using a spoon. Cook for 5 minutes over low heat, or until the water from the sauce has evaporated. Add salt to taste.

Add the sweet potatoes to a serving bowl. Then add the cooked green rice and top with the extras—the black beans, tomato, red cabbage and sliced avocado and sprinkle with the lime juice. Enjoy!

CRISPY TOFU TORTAS

A traditional torta is a Mexican sandwich on a white roll that's usually grilled or toasted in a press. Typically, tortas are garnished with jalapeño, tomato, onion and avocado. For vegetarians, tortas are usually off limits because they contain some kind of meat, such as pork or beef. We wanted to put a healthy spin on this traditional food by using crispy tofu as the base instead of red meat. The result is an absolutely refreshing, mouthwatering torta that literally took our breath away. It's chock-full of about 1 cup (227 g) of fresh veggies as well, making it perfect for a vegetarian reboot.

Vegan / 30 minutes or less

Serves: 1 / **Calories:** 426 / **Carbohydrates:** 46 g / **Protein:** 24 g / **Fat:** 18 g

- ½ cup (126 g) cooked crispy tofu or ¼ (16-oz [454-g]) block extra-firm tofu
- ¼ cup (18 g) shredded cabbage
- ¼ cup (28 g) grated carrot
- ½ shallot
- 4 cherry tomatoes
- ⅛ jalapeño
- 1 tbsp plus 2 tsp (15 ml) lime juice, divided
- Pinch of salt
- ½ avocado
- ⅛ tsp garlic powder
- One 100% whole-wheat roll
- 2 slices tomato

If you are doing this recipe as part of the sample 1-week meal plan, you should have leftover tofu from the Crispy Black Pepper Tofu with Green Beans recipe on page 173. If not, follow the tofu preparation directions in the Tofu Banh Mi Sandwich recipe on page 99 or in the Spicy Thai Tofu Tacos with Peanut Sauce recipe on page 150.

In a bowl, combine the shredded cabbage and grated carrot. Set aside.

To make the pico de gallo, dice the shallot, cherry tomatoes and jalapeño (if you don't want this too spicy, remove any seeds from the jalapeño and cut out the white flesh) and add to a bowl. Sprinkle with 1 tablespoon of the lime juice and a pinch of salt.

For the avocado mash, using a fork, mash the avocado and remaining 2 teaspoons (10 ml) lime juice in a bowl, then sprinkle with salt and add the garlic powder.

Slice the roll in half and toast each side in the toaster or oven. Spread the avocado mixture on each half of the toasted bread. Then add the crispy tofu, cabbage mixture, pico de gallo and sliced tomatoes to the bottom slice. Add the top half of bread, cut in half and enjoy!

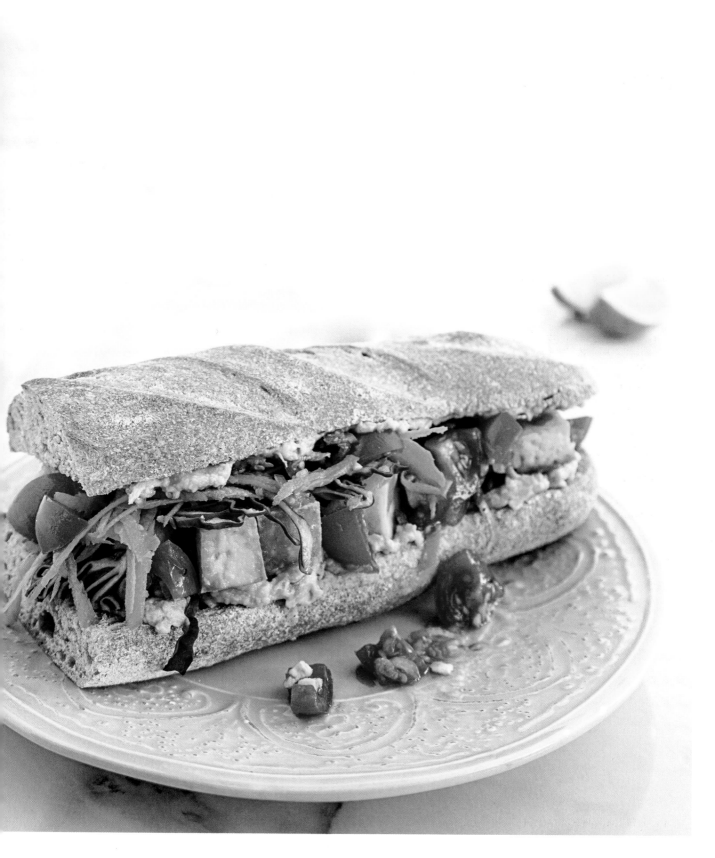

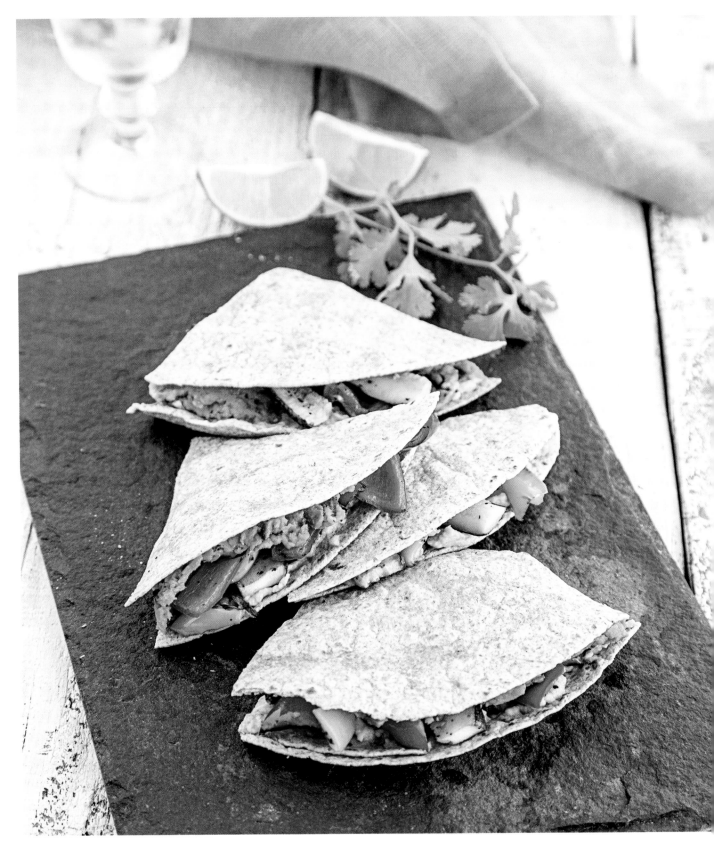

VEGAN AVOCADO SWEET POTATO QUESADILLA

Who would have thought that you could replace cheese with sweet potatoes and actually elevate the flavor? (Why, we did, of course!) The thing is, we love cheese, but as lactose-intolerant chicas, too much of it can hurt our tummies. That's why we like to experiment with cheese alternatives from time to time. This recipe is also a vitamin A and C powerhouse, thanks to all of the vegetables involved here.

Vegan

Serves: 1 (Calculation based on 1 tsp vegetable oil) / **Calories:** 555 / **Carbohydrates:** 73 g / **Protein:** 12 g / **Fat:** 24 g

- ½ **sweet potato**
- 1–2 tsp (5–10 ml) **olive oil, divided**
- ⅛ **red bell pepper**
- ⅛ **yellow bell pepper**
- ¼ **zucchini**
- **Salt to taste**
- ½ **avocado**
- **Juice of ¼ lime**
- 2 (8" [20.5-cm]) 100% whole-wheat tortillas

Preheat the oven to 425°F (218°C). Line a baking sheet with parchment paper.

Chop the sweet potato into cubes, then toss with 1 teaspoon olive oil to coat. Spread on one side of the prepared baking sheet and roast for 10 minutes.

Chop the red and yellow peppers and slice the zucchini lengthwise. Toss the vegetables in a bowl with 1 teaspoon olive oil and salt. When the sweet potatoes have finished the first 10 minutes of roasting, remove from the oven and spread the peppers and zucchini on the other side of the baking sheet. Roast for 10 to 15 minutes longer, or until all the vegetables are tender.

Mash the roasted sweet potatoes with a fork or pulse in a food processor, sprinkle with a pinch of salt and set aside.

Meanwhile, add the avocado and lime juice to a bowl, then mash until the avocado is somewhat creamy. Set aside.

Warm both tortillas in a cast-iron skillet over medium-high heat for 15 seconds on each side. Add the avocado mixture to one tortilla, then top with the cooked peppers. Spread the mashed sweet potato over the second tortilla, then place atop the avocado tortilla, sweet potato side down. Heat in the skillet over medium-high heat for 30 seconds on each side. Cut into fourths and serve.

> ### Note
> If you choose to microwave the sweet potato to save time, you don't need to chop it. Simply wet the sweet potato, puncture holes in it with a fork and wrap it in a damp paper towel. Microwave on high power for 3 to 5 minutes, or until soft. Let cool for 2 to 3 minutes and then remove the skin. Mash the peeled sweet potato with a fork or pulse in the food processor and sprinkle with salt.

SUN-DRIED TOMATO AND BASIL QUESADILLA

Mexican food is one of our favorite types of cuisine, mostly because it tastes great, but also because it's ridiculously easy to make vegetarian. From tacos to taquitos to quesadillas, the varieties are pretty much endless. In this quesadilla recipe, we take a classic Mexican dish and add an Italian twist. The spinach and cheese will keep you full for a long time and, most importantly, the fusion of flavors will make your taste buds happy.

30 minutes or less

Serves: 1 / **Calories:** 544 / **Carbohydrates:** 52 g / **Protein:** 24 g / **Fat:** 26 g

- 1 tsp vegetable oil
- 1 cup (30 g) chopped raw spinach
- 1 clove garlic, minced
- 2 (8" [20.5-cm]) 100% whole-wheat tortillas
- ½ cup (57 g) shredded mozzarella cheese
- 8 basil leaves, chopped
- 2 tsp (2 g) chopped sun-dried tomatoes
- ¼ cup (61 g) 2% Greek yogurt (optional)

Heat the oil in a skillet over medium heat, add the spinach and garlic and sauté until the spinach is wilted (but still bright green) and the garlic is fragrant. This usually takes 2 to 5 minutes.

While the spinach is cooking, warm up the tortillas by heating them in a skillet over medium-high heat for about 15 seconds on each side. Add the shredded cheese to one tortilla, then add the spinach sauté and fresh chopped basil. Top this with the sun-dried tomatoes. Cover with the remaining tortilla and cook in the cast iron skillet until the cheese is melted and the tortilla is crisp—this usually takes about 30 seconds per side. Keep in mind you'll have to flip this one or two times as needed. When the quesadilla is done, remove it from the pan and cut it into fourths. If you want a dipping sauce, serve it with ¼ cup (61 g) of 2% Greek yogurt instead of sour cream (more protein, less calories).

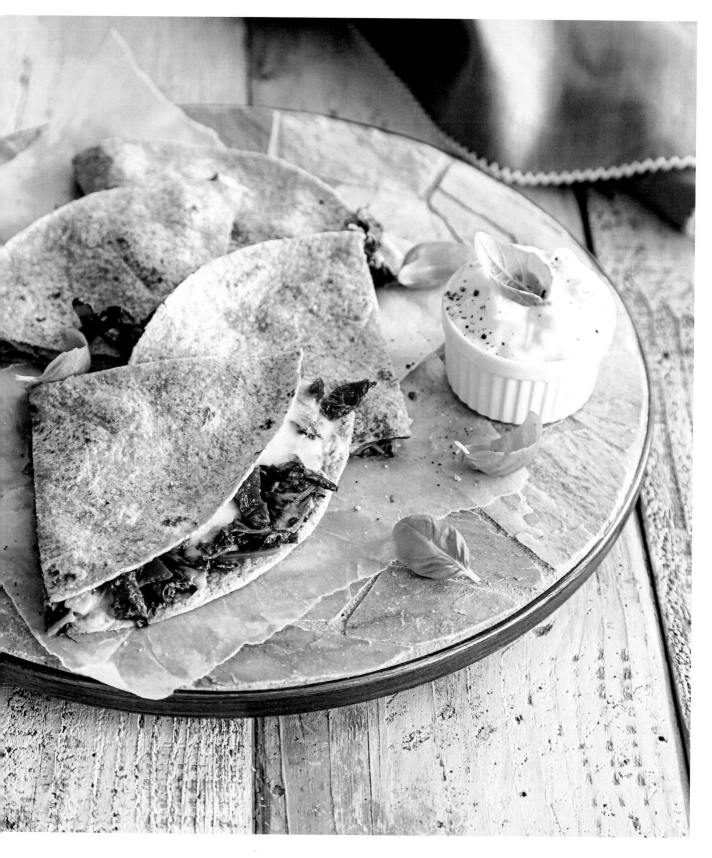

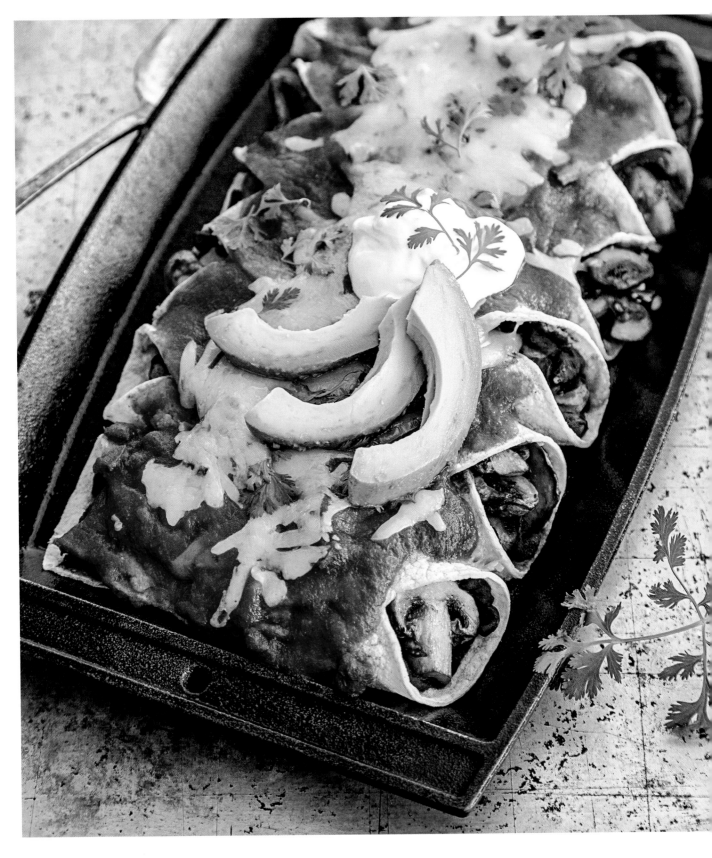

MUSHROOM BLACK BEAN ENCHILADAS

As much as we love enchiladas, we sometimes feel heavy and fatigued after eating them. We decided to create a light and mouthwatering vegetarian rendition, packed with nourishing goodness. One of our main stuffing ingredients is button mushrooms, which don't get the shine they deserve. They are a good source of B vitamins, including riboflavin, pantothenic acid and niacin. Mushrooms are extremely flexible in the kitchen and soak up the flavors and spices they are cooked in. Using them as an enchilada stuffing is going to leave you thinking of other ways to incorporate them into your dishes!

Gluten-free (if using gluten-free soy sauce)

Serves: 2

Per Serving / **Calories:** 545 / **Carbohydrates:** 74 g / **Protein:** 21 g / **Fat:** 19 g

- 1 tbsp (15 ml) olive oil
- ½ tsp brown sugar
- ½ onion, chopped
- 4 cups (288 g) sliced button mushrooms
- ½ tsp soy sauce
- 1 cup (245 g) tomato sauce
- 1 tbsp (8 g) red chili powder
- 1 tsp garlic powder
- 1 tsp ground cumin, divided
- 1 jalapeño pepper, seeded and chopped
- Salt to taste
- 1 cup (185 g) cooked black beans
- 6 corn tortillas
- ¼ cup (28 g) shredded pepper Jack cheese
- ¼ avocado, sliced
- 1 cup (50 g) fresh cilantro
- 1 tbsp (14 g) sour cream

Preheat the oven to 350°F (177°C). Have a medium-sized 8 x 8-inch (20.5 x 20.5-cm) baking dish on hand.

Heat the olive oil in a skillet over medium heat and add the brown sugar. Cook for about 2 minutes, or until the sugar starts to get darker in color. Add the onion and sauté for another 2 minutes. Add the sliced mushrooms and soy sauce and cover with the lid. Cook for 5 to 7 minutes or until the mushrooms are a deep-brown color, stirring midway through. Remove from the heat and set aside.

To make the enchilada sauce, combine the tomato sauce, red chili powder, garlic powder, ½ teaspoon of the cumin and the jalapeño in a pot. Cook over medium heat for 10 minutes, stirring occasionally, then add salt to taste.

While the sauce is cooking, mash the black beans with the remaining ½ teaspoon cumin and add salt to taste.

If your tortillas are not very soft, heat them for 2 to 3 minutes in a microwave or in a pan over low heat to make them more pliable. When the tortillas are soft, spread one-sixth of the black bean paste onto each tortilla. Then spread each with one-sixth of the sautéed mushrooms and top each with the shredded cheese. Roll each tortilla up and place in the baking dish. Pour three-fourths of the enchilada sauce over the rolled tortillas. Pop the dish into the oven and bake for 20 minutes. The enchiladas are done when the tortilla edges are lightly crisped, and the cheese has melted.

Remove them from the oven, pour the remaining enchilada sauce over the dish and top with the sliced avocado, fresh cilantro and a dollop of sour cream.

ROASTED RED PEPPER COCONUT CAULIFLOWER

This creamy cauliflower is the perfect case for showing how versatile and delicious vegetables can be. Don't let the lack of color in cauliflower fool you. One cup (124 g) of this super vegetable has more than 70 percent of your daily vitamin C needs. Cauliflower is also a good source of choline, which is important for brain function and memory. Paired with brown rice, it makes for an incredibly satisfying and nutritious meal!

Gluten-free (if using gluten-free soy sauce) / Vegan

Serves: 3

Per Serving / Calories: 400 / **Carbohydrates:** 65 g / **Protein:** 10 g / **Fat:** 12 g

RICE

- 2½ cups (592 ml) water
- 1 cup (190 g) uncooked brown rice
- Salt to taste

CAULIFLOWER

- 1 medium head cauliflower
- 1 large red bell pepper
- ½ onion, chopped
- 3 cloves garlic
- ½ cup (120 ml) coconut milk
- 1 cup (237 ml) water
- 1 tbsp (15 ml) soy sauce
- Salt and cayenne pepper to taste

For the rice, bring the water to a boil in a pot. Add the brown rice and cook over low to medium heat for 35 to 40 minutes, or until the rice is soft and tender. Add salt to taste.

Preheat the oven to 400°F (204°C). Line a baking sheet with parchment paper.

For the cauliflower, remove any outer leaves and slice off the stem from the base. Then cut the cauliflower into small 1 x 1-inch (2.5 x 2.5-cm) florets. Set aside.

Cut the stem off the red bell pepper, slice it in half and remove the seeds and the white fibrous flesh from the insides. Spread on the prepared baking sheet and roast it for 30 minutes, until tender. Remove it from the oven and let it cool slightly. Add it to a food processor, along with the onion and garlic, and process into a paste.

Combine the pepper paste, coconut milk and water in a pot over medium heat and cook for 5 minutes. Then add the cauliflower florets and soy sauce and cook over low heat, with the lid on, for 15 minutes, or until the cauliflower is tender. Add salt and cayenne pepper to taste. Serve over the brown rice.

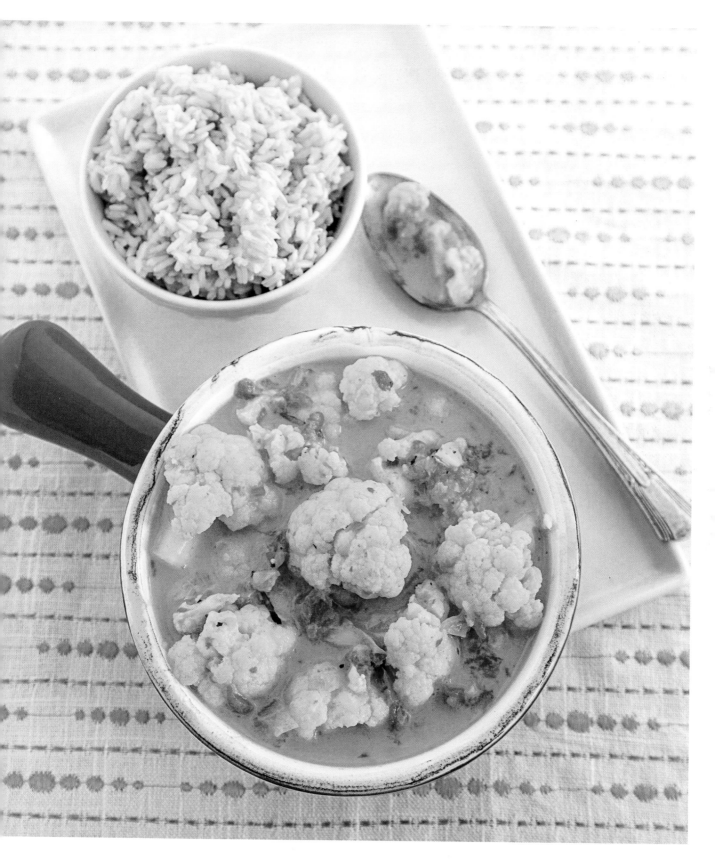

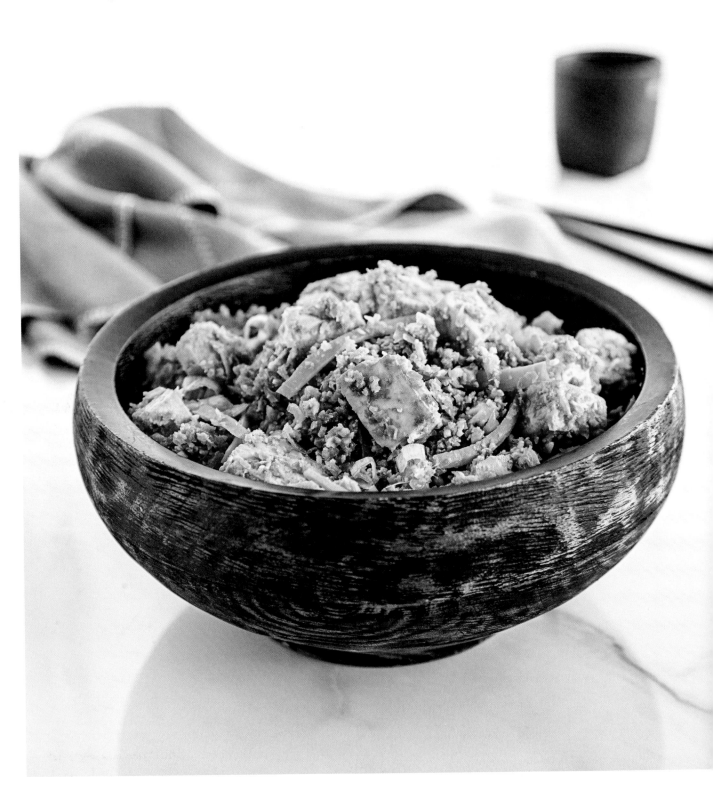

EASY TOFU CAULIFLOWER FRIED RICE

When we first heard about cauliflower rice, we thought it sounded too good to be true. And then we tried it. Um, amazing. Seriously, if you are looking for an easy way to sneak in more vegetables without even trying, this is definitely it. This recipe is as delicious as it is healthy. Cauliflower is a vitamin C powerhouse (meeting 73 percent of your needs for the day), which gives it special antioxidant powers. It's also a great source of vitamin K, folate, B_6 and more than ten other vitamins and minerals. This recipe is low carb and full of protein to boot. Enjoy half now and store half in an airtight container in the refrigerator for later.

Gluten-free (if using gluten-free soy sauce) / 30 minutes or less

Serves: 2

Per Serving / Calories: 391 / **Carbohydrates:** 29 g / **Protein:** 25 g / **Fat:** 21 g

· 1 head cauliflower

· 1½ tsp (7.5 ml) sesame oil

· 2 cloves garlic, chopped

· 1 tsp minced fresh ginger

· 10 baby carrots, thinly sliced

· ½ (16-oz [454-g]) block extra-firm tofu

· 2 scallions, chopped

· 1½ tsp (7.5 ml) soy sauce

· 2 eggs

· Salt and pepper to taste

Remove the leaves and cut out the core from the cauliflower. Chop the cauliflower into small florets—this makes for easy pulsing. Toss in a food processor and pulse until the cauliflower is small and grainy looking—basically resembling rice. Note: Depending on the size and power of your food processor, you may need to do this in a few batches.

Heat the sesame oil in a pan over medium heat. Add the garlic, ginger, carrots and tofu, stir to blend and cook for 3 to 5 minutes, or until it starts to smell delicious. Add the cauliflower, then scallions and soy sauce; sauté for 5 additional minutes. Lower the heat, push all the ingredients to the side of the pan to create a well in the middle and add the eggs. Let them cook for about 30 to 60 seconds and then stir gently with the rest of the ingredients until the eggs are fully cooked. Season with salt and pepper to taste.

THAI BASIL EGGPLANT WITH TOFU AND BROWN RICE

If you're looking for a vegetable that will fill you up, eggplant is definitely it. One cup (82 g) meets 10 percent of your daily fiber needs, while providing just 30 calories. Eggplant is such a fun ingredient to cook with because there are so many ways it can be incorporated into dishes. It acts as a sponge, soaking up all of the flavors it's cooked in. In this recipe, the result is a rich and savory dish, with delicate undertones of sweet basil.

Gluten-free (if using gluten-free soy sauce) / Vegan

Serves: 2
Per Serving / Calories: 434 / **Carbohydrates:** 55 g / **Protein:** 15 g / **Fat:** 19 g

RICE

- 1½ cups (355 ml) water
- ½ cup (93 g) uncooked brown rice
- Salt to taste

TOFU

- ½ (16-oz [454-g]) block firm tofu
- 1 tbsp (17 g) roasted red chile paste
- 1 tsp garlic powder
- 1 tsp rice vinegar
- 1 tbsp (15 ml) olive oil
- 1 red bell pepper, seeded and sliced into strips
- 1 green bell pepper, seeded and sliced into strips
- ½ medium red onion, sliced into rounds
- 2 cups (164 g) cubed eggplant
- 1 tsp soy sauce
- ¼ cup (11 g) thinly sliced fresh basil
- Salt to taste
- Sriracha to taste (optional)

For the rice, bring the water to a boil in a pot, add the rice and cook for 30 to 35 minutes, or until tender. Season with salt to taste.

For the tofu, using your hands or a paper towel, press the water out of the tofu block until there is no more water dripping from it. Cut it into 1-inch (2.5-cm) cubes. Place the tofu cubes in a bowl and sprinkle with the chile paste, garlic powder and rice vinegar. Using your hands, massage the marinade ingredients into the tofu so that all the cubes are coated. Let the tofu marinate in the bowl for at least 20 minutes.

Heat the olive oil in a pan over medium heat, add the peppers and onion and sauté for 2 to 3 minutes. Add the cubed eggplant, drizzle the soy sauce over the eggplant, cover with a lid and cook for 10 minutes without stirring. When the eggplant has softened and has turned a deep brown color, add the marinated tofu and stir the ingredients well. Cook for 8 to 10 minutes over low to medium heat, with the lid off, stirring occasionally. Top with fresh basil and add salt to taste. You can also drizzle with Sriracha sauce if you want an extra kick of spice.

Serve with the rice.

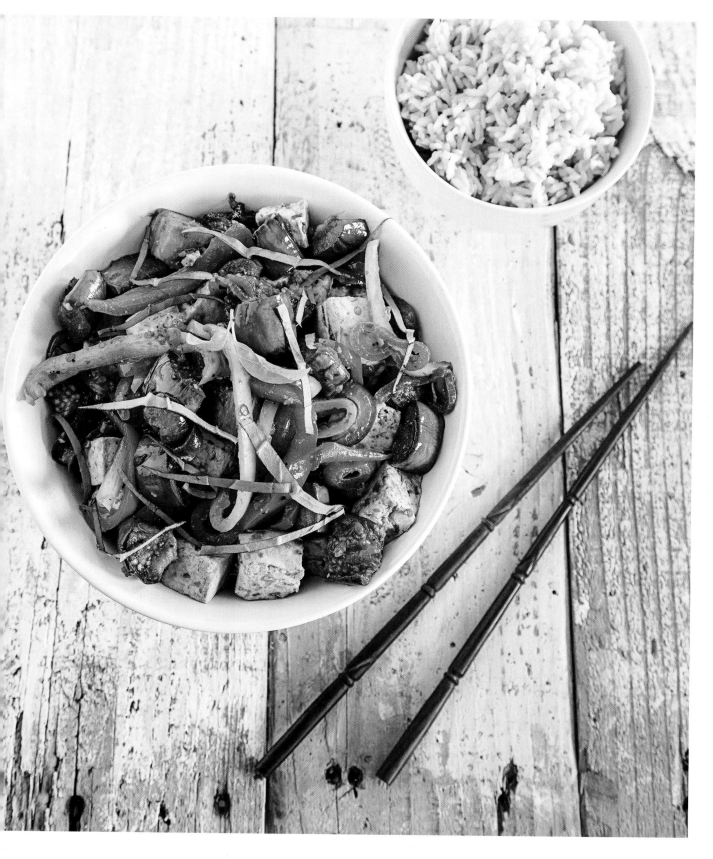

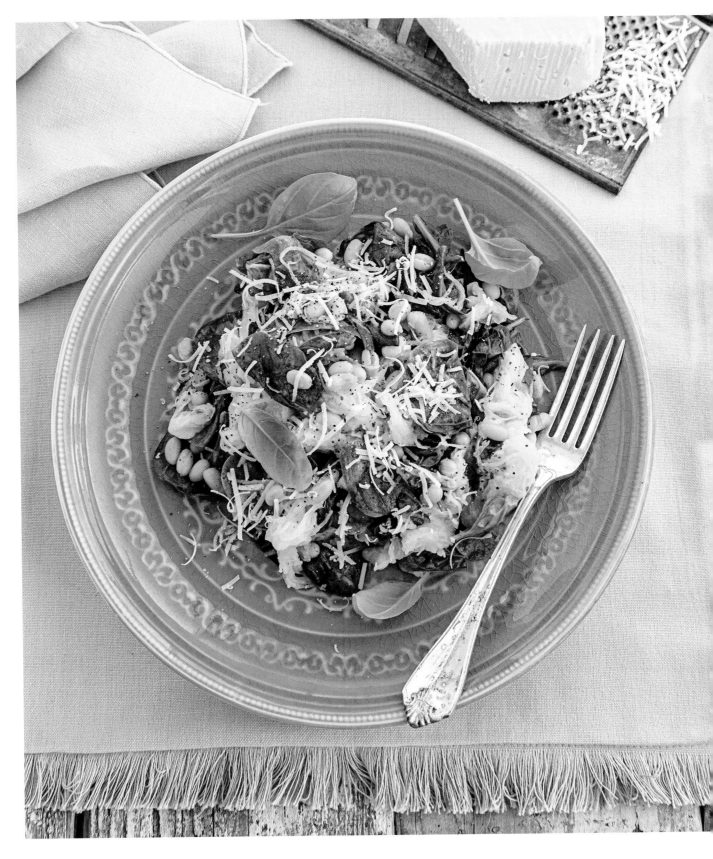

ROASTED GARLIC WHITE BEAN SPAGHETTI SQUASH

Spaghetti squash can be used to create lighter alternatives to pasta dishes. It has just 42 calories per serving—a fraction of what is in traditional pasta. It also has just 10 grams of carbohydrates per serving, making it a great option for people who have challenges controlling their blood sugar. The roasted garlic and white beans add creamy, savory notes to the dish. Topped with the sweetness of the fresh basil? Absolutely everything.

Gluten-free

Serves: 2

Per Serving / Calories: 375 **/ Carbohydrates:** 43 g **/ Protein:** 18 g **/ Fat:** 19 g

- 1 medium spaghetti squash
- 1 cup (237 ml) water
- 1 head garlic
- 1¼ tsp (6 ml) olive oil, divided
- 1 cup (179 g) cooked white beans
- 3 cups (90 g) raw spinach
- 2 tbsp (13 g) grated Parmesan
- Salt and black pepper to taste
- ¼ cup (11 g) fresh basil

Preheat the oven to 400°F (204°C).

Using a very sharp knife, slice the spaghetti squash lengthwise in half. Using a spoon, scoop out all the seeds. Place in a baking dish, cut sides up, and add the water to the bottom of the baking dish. Set aside.

Trim the top of the garlic head, place it on a piece of aluminum foil and drizzle it with ¼ teaspoon of the olive oil. Wrap the garlic with the foil. Bake both the garlic and the spaghetti squash for 30 to 40 minutes, or until you can easily stick a fork through the firm squash flesh. Allow the squash to cool. Using a fork, pull the squash flesh up from the peel, creating spaghetti-like strands. Scoop the strands into a bowl and set aside. Remove the garlic cloves from the skin and set aside.

Heat the remaining 1 teaspoon olive oil in a skillet over medium heat, add the roasted garlic and white beans and cook for 1 minute, then add the spinach and spaghetti squash "noodles." Cover the pan and cook until the spinach has wilted, 2 to 3 minutes. Mix all of the ingredients well and cook for another 5 minutes over low heat, with the lid on. Remove from the heat, add the Parmesan, season with salt and black pepper to taste and finish by topping with the fresh basil.

PEPPER JACK ZUCCHINI QUESADILLA

As outpatient dietitians, we both teach nutrition classes for kids and adults. Parents often tell us that their kids hate all vegetables, and getting away with anything green on the plate might be a bigger challenge than getting to the moon. In her Eat Smart, Healthy Start program, Jess cooks healthy recipes with kids to help them learn how to make delicious meals and snacks. One of the most popular recipes is this pepper Jack zucchini quesadilla. The kids love getting to carve out faces in the tortilla (you don't have to do that here—unless you want to!) and they get to grate the cheese themselves. The recipe can be as simple as three ingredients (zucchini, cheese, tortilla) or as elaborate as you want to make it. We hope you love it.

30 minutes or less

Serves: 1 / **Calories:** 551 / **Carbohydrates:** 60 g / **Protein:** 25 g / **Fat:** 22 g

SALSA

- 5 cherry tomatoes
- ⅛ jalapeño, seeded
- Small handful of cilantro
- ½ shallot
- Juice of ¼ lime
- Salt and pepper to taste

QUESADILLA

- 1 clove garlic
- ¼ zucchini
- 1 tsp vegetable oil
- 2 (8" [20.5-cm]) 100% whole-wheat tortillas
- ⅓ cup (37 g) shredded pepper Jack cheese

"SOUR CREAM"

- ⅓ cup (81 g) 2% Greek yogurt

For the salsa, chop the cherry tomatoes, jalapeño, cilantro and shallot. Toss the mixture in a bowl and drizzle with the lime juice. Add freshly ground salt and pepper to taste. Set aside.

For the quesadilla, mince the garlic and grate the zucchini. Heat the vegetable oil over medium heat, add the garlic, then the zucchini, and cook for 3 to 5 minutes, or until fragrant. While the zucchini is cooking, warm up the tortillas in a skillet over medium-high heat for about 15 seconds on each side. Sprinkle the shredded cheese on one tortilla, then add the zucchini sauté. Cover with the remaining tortilla. Cook over medium-high heat until the cheese is melted and the tortilla is crisp, about 30 seconds per side. Keep in mind you'll have to flip this one or two times as needed. Serve with the salsa and "sour cream."

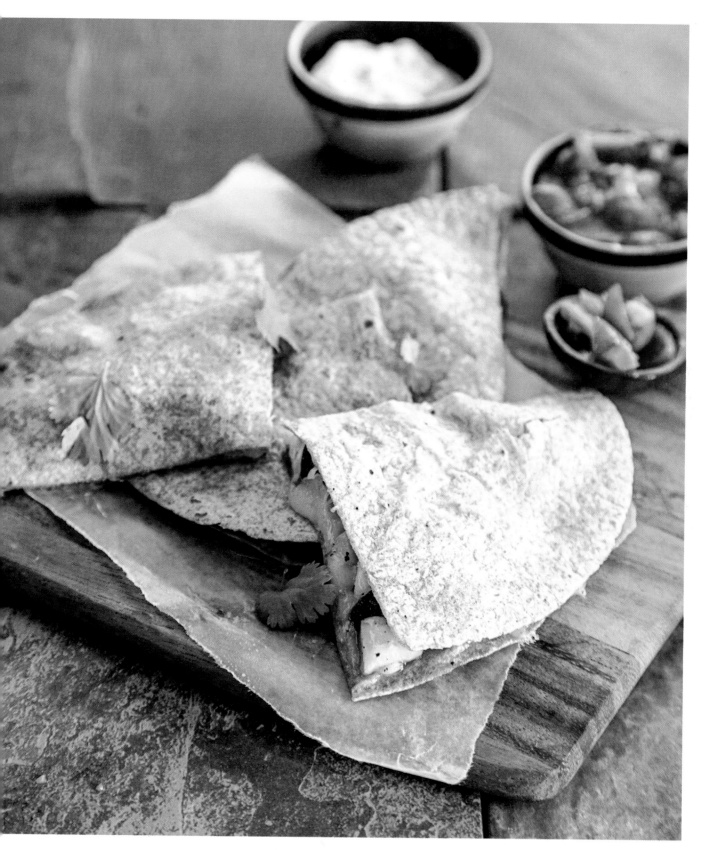

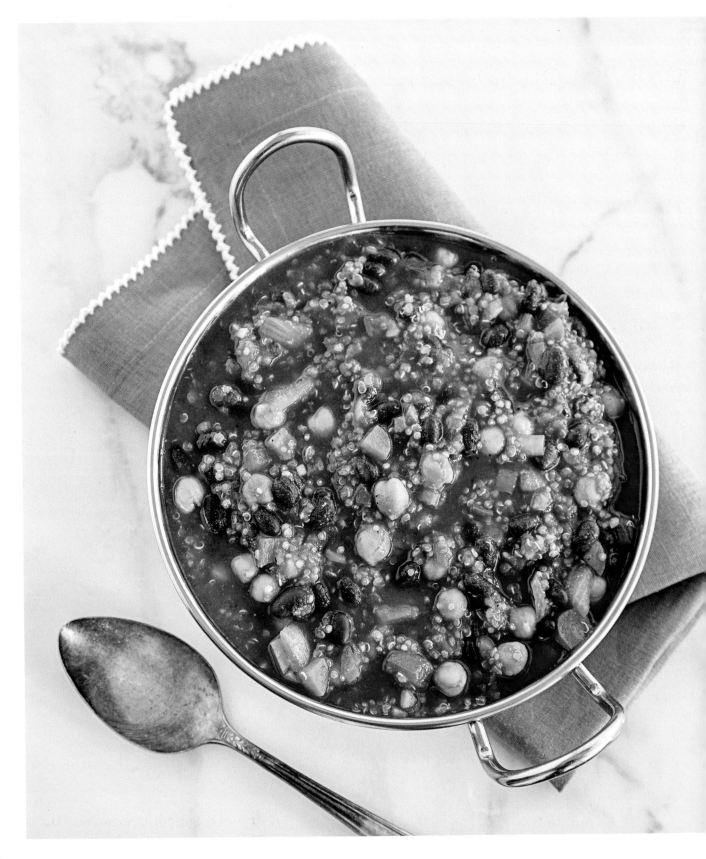

ONE-POT QUINOA CHILI

This savory black bean and chickpea quinoa chili is going to add so much life to your lunch hour. It's the result of combining really amazing ingredients together in a pot and letting heat work its magic. Besides providing all of the essential amino acids, quinoa is a good source of folate, magnesium and manganese. It can be incorporated into stews like this one, or it can be used in salads, baked goods, soups and so much more!

Gluten-free / Vegan

Serves: 4

Per Serving / Calories: 449 / **Carbohydrates:** 71 g / **Protein:** 22 g / **Fat:** 8 g

- ½ medium onion, chopped
- 1 large tomato, cubed
- ½ medium red bell pepper, seeded and chopped
- 3 cloves garlic, minced
- ¼ cup (32 g) chopped carrot
- 1 jalapeño, seeded and chopped
- 1 tbsp (15 ml) olive oil
- 2½ cups (592 ml) water
- 2 cups (490 g) tomato sauce
- 1 (15.5-oz [358-g]) can black beans, drained and rinsed
- 1 (15.5-oz [358-g]) can chickpeas, drained and rinsed
- ½ cup (85 g) uncooked quinoa
- 1 tsp ground cumin
- 1 tsp chili powder
- Salt and cayenne pepper to taste

In a bowl, combine the onion, tomato, red bell pepper, garlic, carrot and jalapeño. Mix them together with a spoon.

Heat the olive oil in a large pot over medium heat, add the onion mixture and sauté for 5 minutes. When those ingredients are fragrant, add the water, tomato sauce, black beans and chickpeas. Stir to combine.

Add the quinoa, cumin and chili powder. Cook for 30 minutes over medium-low heat, stirring every 10 minutes. Add salt and cayenne pepper to taste. Store any leftover chili in the refrigerator and have it as a lunch or dinner option for the week. You can also freeze it for up to 1 month.

STOVETOP TEMPEH RATATOUILLE

Ratatouille is a genius way to enjoy vegetables. The dish is prepared by sautéing different vegetables separately and layering them back into a pot or baking dish. The result is a savory stew that can be served hot or cold. Although we are preparing it as a main dish, it can also be enjoyed as an appetizer or a side. To make this a more complete meal, we added tempeh for an additional boost in calories and protein.

Gluten-free / Vegan

Serves: 2

Per Serving / **Calories:** 488 / **Carbohydrates:** 52 g / **Protein:** 22 g / **Fat:** 23 g

- 6 tsp (30 ml) olive oil, divided into thirds
- 1 medium onion, chopped
- 4 cloves garlic, minced
- 1 red bell pepper, seeded and chopped
- 2 small zucchini, sliced into rounds
- 2 small yellow squash, sliced into rounds
- 4 cups (328 g) cubed eggplant
- 4 medium tomatoes, chopped
- 2 bay leaves
- 4 sprigs fresh thyme
- 1 cup (166 g) cubed tempeh
- 2 tsp (4 g) dried oregano
- Salt and cayenne pepper to taste

Heat 2 teaspoons (10 ml) of the olive oil in a large pot over medium heat. Add the onion, garlic and pepper and sauté for 5 minutes, stirring occasionally. Remove from the pot and transfer to a bowl.

Heat another 2 teaspoons (10 ml) of olive oil in the pot and add the zucchini and squash rounds. Sauté for 7 to 8 minutes, stirring occasionally, until the zucchini and squash rounds have browned on the edges. Add them to the same bowl with the other sautéed ingredients.

Heat the remaining 2 teaspoons (10 ml) of olive oil, add the cubed eggplant and sauté for 10 minutes, stirring occasionally. Add that to the bowl as well.

Finally, add the tomatoes, bay leaves and thyme to the pot and cook for 7 minutes, stirring occasionally. Now add all of the vegetables from the bowl back into the pot with the tomatoes, add the tempeh and oregano and cook for 10 to 12 minutes over low heat. Remove the bay leaves and add salt and cayenne pepper to taste. Enjoy!

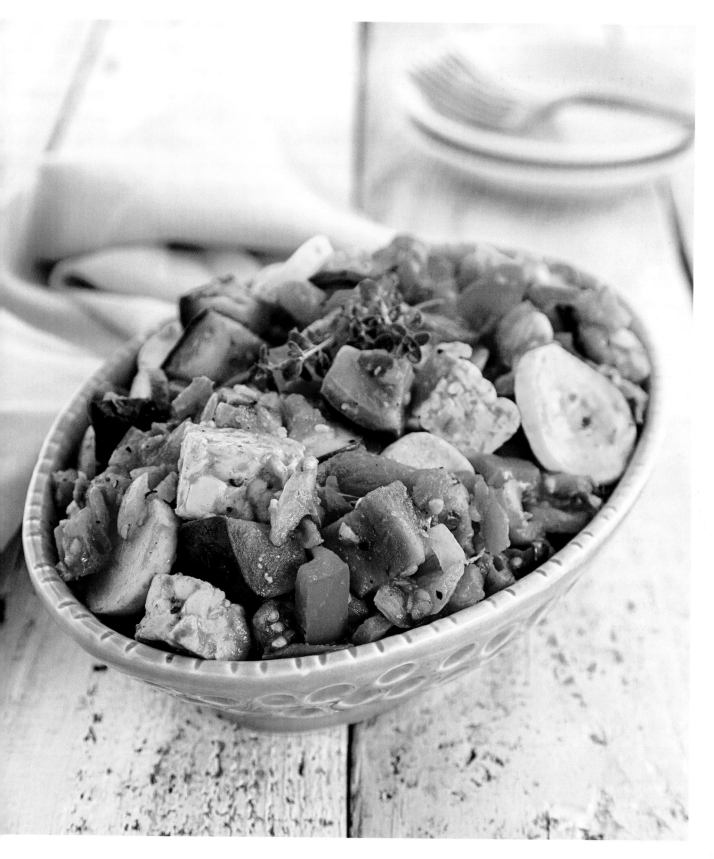

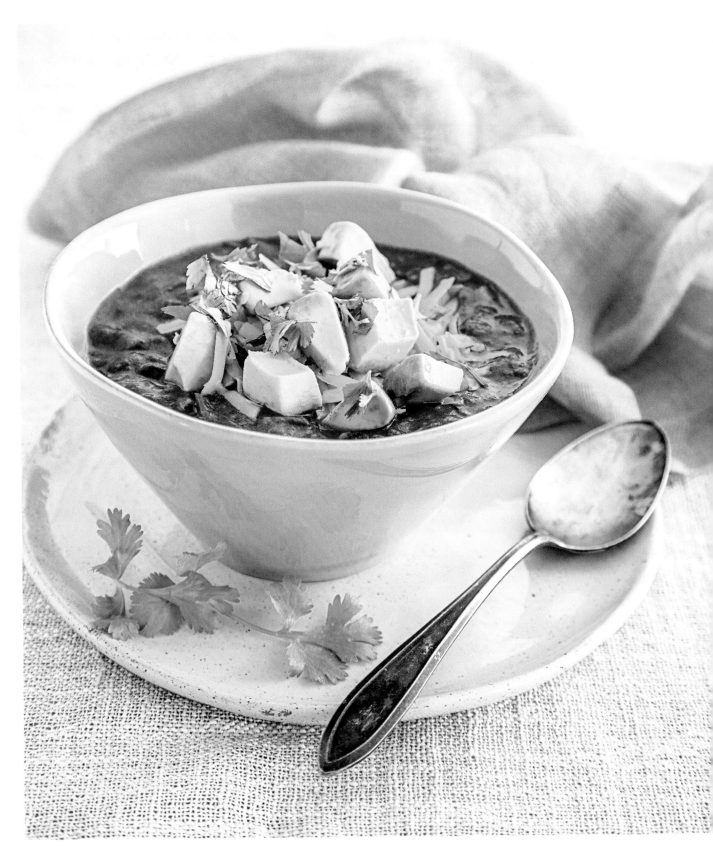

DELICIOUS DINNERS TO END YOUR DAY RIGHT

We intentionally added our quicker and simpler recipes into this section, because the last thing we want you to do is spend hours in the kitchen after a long day. Recipes like our Garlic Artichoke Pita Pizza (page 170), Black Olive Grilled Cheese (page 177) and Eggplant Gyro (page 186) all take well under 30 minutes to prepare and will leave you feeling satisfied and content. For those of you who have weight loss in mind, make dinner one of your lighter meals, since we tend to be less active as the day closes out. Also aim to eat dinners three hours before bedtime. This may help prevent acid reflux, improve sleep and ensure you are hungry for breakfast in the morning. On your less busy days, you have the option of preparing more elaborate dinners that yield multiple servings, like our Vegan Clam Chowder (page 149) or the mouthwatering Tomato Split Pea Soup with Coconut Collard Greens (page 145). Leave the leftovers in the fridge or freezer, and when you come home ready for a quick meal, simply reheat and enjoy. Happy dining!

SIMPLE BLACK BEAN ENCHILADA SOUP

Soup + enchiladas. Two things that sound like they don't go together, but their union breeds a food baby so perfect, you'll kick yourself for not having thought of it before. Flavor aside, perhaps the best part is that this soup is ridiculously easy to make. The whole recipe—including the homemade enchilada sauce (!)—will take you 20 minutes to prepare, tops. We made sure to include black beans because they give you protein and a healthy dose of fiber (7.5 grams per ½ cup [93 g], to be exact). We top this soup off with a bit of cilantro, which studies suggest may help control blood sugar and prevent free radical production, though more research is needed. Either way, this soup will rock your socks and warm your soul, so let's get the party started.

Gluten-free (if using gluten-free vegetable stock) / 30 minutes or less

Serves: 2

Per serving / Calories: 582 / **Carbohydrates:** 49 g / **Protein:** 17 g / **Fat:** 37 g

ENCHILADA SAUCE

- 4 tsp (20 ml) vegetable oil
- 2 tsp (5 g) cornstarch
- ⅔ cup (160 ml) vegetable stock
- 2 tsp (5 g) chili powder
- ½ tsp garlic powder
- ½ tsp ground cumin
- Salt to taste

ENCHILADA SOUP

- 2 tsp (10 ml) vegetable oil
- ¼ red onion, diced
- 3 cloves garlic, minced
- 2 tsp (5 g) cornstarch
- 2 cups (470 ml) vegetable stock
- 1 cup (185 g) cooked black beans

- 2 roma tomatoes, diced
- ½ cup (56.6 g) shredded cheddar cheese
- ⅓ avocado, chopped
- Small handful of cilantro, chopped

(continued)

SIMPLE BLACK BEAN ENCHILADA SOUP (CONTINUED)

For the enchilada sauce, combine the oil, cornstarch, veggie stock and spices in a bowl and stir well. Set aside.

For the soup, heat the oil in a pot over medium-low heat. Add the onion and cook for 2 to 3 minutes, then add the garlic and cook for 2 minutes longer, or until it starts smelling divine.

Add the cornstarch and stir well to coat the onion and garlic. Then add the veggie stock and stir, stir, stir. Add the cooked black beans (we used canned) and the tomatoes to the soup. Lower the heat to a simmer and let it cook/thicken for an additional 5 or so minutes. Mix in your enchilada sauce and top the soup with the shredded cheese, avocado and cilantro.

ASIAN STIR-FRY WITH CRISPY TOFU

If you're like many people, you may be wondering: Is soy safe to eat? A lot of people fear soy because they've heard that the phytoestrogen content will wreak havoc in the body (namely causing breast cancer in women and making men grow breasts). Well, we scoured the research—specifically research on humans—and it led us to two conclusions: 1) soy has an insignificant effect on breast cancer, and some studies have even shown that it can actually protect against certain types of cancer and heart disease, and 2) soy is relatively new to us in the United States, but there are various countries in Asia that have been eating soy within the context of a traditional diet forever, and there has been no evidence of harm. As dietitians, we believe that eating organic, minimally processed soy (which includes tofu) is absolutely fine in moderation. So let's get this recipe started, shall we?

Gluten-free (if using gluten-free soy sauce) / Vegan

Serves: 2
Per Serving / Calories: 517 **/ Carbohydrates:** 55 g **/ Protein:** 23 g **/ Fat:** 25 g

STIR-FRY

· ½ (16-oz [454-g]) block extra-firm tofu

· 2 tsp (10 ml) vegetable oil, divided in half

· 1 cup (195 g) cooked brown rice or ⅓ cup (65 g) uncooked rice and ⅔ cup (160 ml) water

· ⅔ red onion, thinly sliced

· 1 red bell pepper, seeded and sliced

· 1 green bell pepper, seeded and sliced

· 1 tsp chopped fresh ginger

· 2 cloves garlic, minced

· ¼ cup (25 g) cilantro, chopped

PEANUT SAUCE

· 3 tsp (16 g) creamy peanut butter

· 4 tsp (20 ml) water

· 1 tsp rice vinegar

· 1 tsp soy sauce

· 1 clove garlic

· 1 (½-inch [3.9-cm]) piece of fresh ginger, peeled

· 1 tsp toasted sesame seed oil

· Salt and pepper to taste

(continued)

ASIAN STIR-FRY WITH CRISPY TOFU (CONTINUED)

For the stir-fry, remove the tofu from the package and wrap it in a clean towel. Use half of the block for this recipe and save the remaining half for later by submerging it in water (in an airtight container) and storing it in the refrigerator for 3 to 5 days. Place the towel-wrapped tofu in a glass pan, then put something heavy on top. The idea is to press all of the water out of the tofu for up to 4 hours. When the tofu is drained, cut it into small cubes (about ½ x ½-inch [1.3 x 1.3-cm]).

Preheat the oven to 375°F (190°C). Coat a baking sheet with 1 teaspoon of the oil.

Spread the cubed tofu pieces on the prepared baking sheet and bake for 30 minutes, flipping the tofu with a spatula halfway through so it cooks evenly.

If cooking the brown rice from scratch, add the rice and water to a pot and bring it to a boil over medium-high heat. Reduce the heat to medium-low and cover. Simmer until the liquid is completely absorbed, usually about 40 minutes. Let cook and fluff with a fork.

Heat the remaining 1 teaspoon of oil in a skillet (or wok if you have one) over high heat. Add the onion, peppers, ginger and garlic and sauté for 5 to 10 minutes, stirring constantly so that everything cooks evenly without burning.

For the peanut sauce, combine the peanut butter, water, vinegar, soy sauce, garlic, ginger and toasted sesame seed oil in a blender and blend until smooth. Season with salt and pepper to taste. Use half of the peanut sauce now and save the remaining half in an airtight container for Spicy Thai Tofu Tacos with Peanut Sauce (page 150).

Now that we're finished preparing all of the ingredients for this recipe, it's time to plate it. Spoon half of the rice onto each of the 2 plates, then top with half of the stir-fry and tofu. Drizzle the peanut sauce on top and garnish with cilantro. Enjoy!

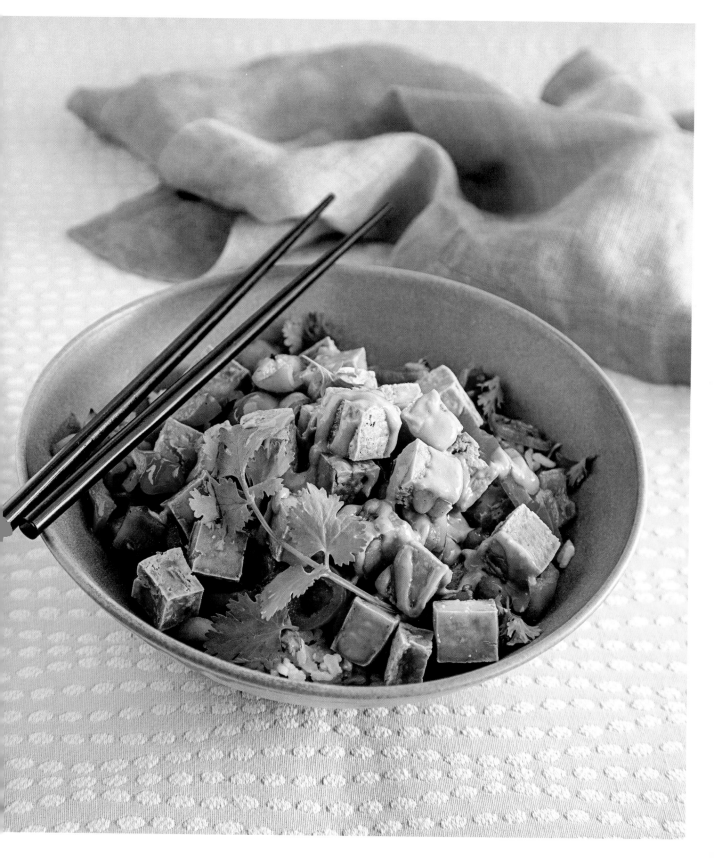

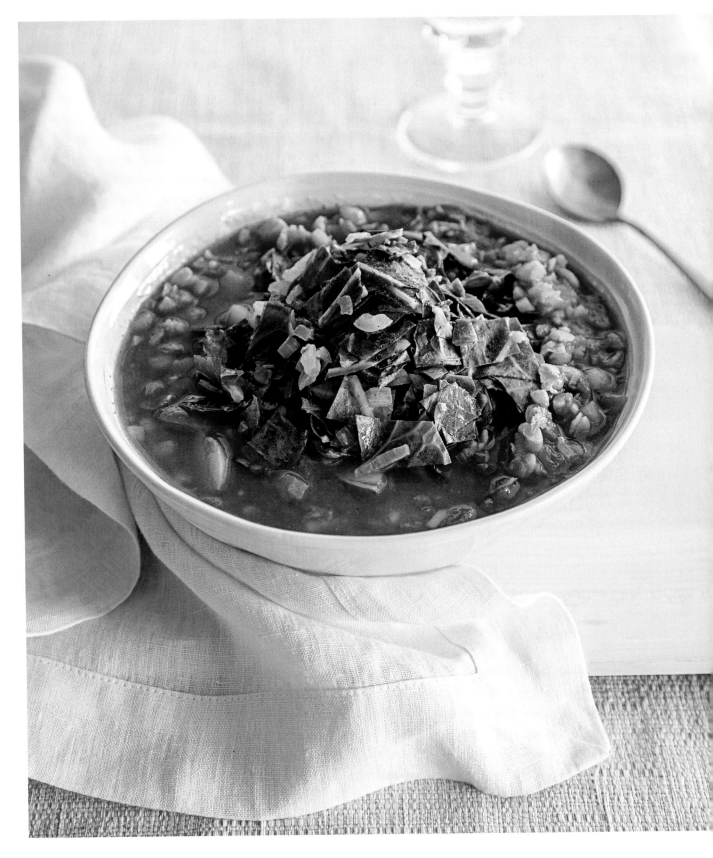

TOMATO SPLIT PEA SOUP WITH COCONUT COLLARD GREENS

Who doesn't love a warm bowl of soup? This hearty split pea soup is topped with savory collards and spiced with a dash of cayenne pepper. Collard greens are often seasoned with pork, but in this recipe we use coconut oil to bring out their richness. Nutritionally speaking, collard greens are a winner; 1 cup (36 g) of this cooked leafy green provides more than 300 percent of your daily vitamin A needs! Collard greens are also an excellent source of calcium and vitamins C and K.

Gluten-free / Vegan

Serves: 2

Per serving / Calories: 512 / **Carbohydrates:** 76 g / **Protein:** 23 g / **Fat:** 15 g

SOUP

· **1 tbsp (14 g) coconut oil**

· **½ medium onion, finely chopped**

· **4 cloves garlic, minced**

· **2 medium tomatoes, cubed**

· **1 tbsp (17 g) tomato paste**

· **4½ cups (1.1 L) water**

· **¾ cup (148 g) dried yellow split peas**

· **1 potato, cubed**

· **Salt and cayenne pepper to taste**

COLLARD GREENS

· **1 tbsp (14 g) coconut oil**

· **1 small onion, finely chopped**

· **1 jalapeño pepper, seeded and minced**

· **3 cups (108 g) finely chopped collard greens**

· **½ tbsp (3 ml) rice vinegar**

For the soup, heat the coconut oil in a large pot and add the onion, garlic and tomatoes. Sauté for 3 to 4 minutes over medium heat or until the ingredients are fragrant, stirring occasionally. Next, add the tomato paste, stir and sauté for another 1 to 2 minutes. Now add the water, split peas and potato, lower the heat to medium-low and cook for 45 minutes, stirring every 10 to 15 minutes.

For the collard greens, heat the coconut oil in a pan over medium heat, add the onion and jalapeño and sauté for 5 minutes or until the ingredients are fragrant, stirring occasionally. Then add the collards and rice vinegar. Cook with the lid on for 5 minutes and set aside when done. The collards should be tender and bright green.

When the soup is finished cooking, add salt and cayenne pepper to taste and top with the collard sauté.

THAI COCONUT CURRY TOFU NOODLE SOUP

The secret to everything Thai is red (or green) curry paste. Seriously. This magic ingredient is jam-packed with flavor and it's super easy to incorporate into many dishes. This Thai noodle soup will make you feel all warm and fuzzy on the inside, especially in the cold winter months. We also added a little heat to this recipe with a dose (you decide how hot you want it) of crushed red pepper flakes, and research suggests that these little buggers may be helpful in fighting inflammation, relieving pain and protecting the heart. Some people even find that chili peppers are great for clearing congestion when they have a cold.

Vegan

Serves: 2
Per Serving / **Calories:** 426 / **Carbohydrates:** 59 g / **Protein:** 18 g / **Fat:** 13 g

---

- ½ (16-oz [454-g]) block extra-firm tofu
- 1 tsp vegetable oil
- 4 oz (113 g) dried udon noodles
- 1 cup (240 ml) light coconut milk
- 2 cups (473 ml) water
- 2 tsp (11 g) Thai red curry paste
- ¼ tsp crushed red pepper flakes, or to taste
- 2 tsp (4 g) curry powder
- Salt to taste
- 4 tsp (8 g) chopped scallion
- 4 tsp (8 g) chopped cilantro

Remove the tofu from the package and wrap it in a clean towel. Use half of the block for this recipe and save the remaining half for later by submerging it in water (in an airtight container) and storing it in the refrigerator for 3 to 5 days. Place the towel-wrapped tofu in a glass pan, then put something heavy on top. The idea is to press all of the water out of the tofu for up to 4 hours. When the tofu is drained, cut it into small cubes (about ½ x ½-inch [1.3 x 1.3-cm]).

Preheat the oven to 375°F (190°C). Coat a baking sheet with the oil.

Spread the cubed tofu on the prepared baking sheet and bake for 30 minutes, flipping the tofu with a spatula halfway through so it cooks evenly.

Next, cook the noodles according to package directions.

Meanwhile, warm the coconut milk and water in a separate pot over medium-high heat for 2 minutes. Add the curry paste, red pepper flakes and curry powder and mix thoroughly. Add the cooked tofu and noodles. Bring to a simmer and cook for about 10 to 15 minutes over medium-low heat. Add salt to taste. Garnish with chopped scallion and cilantro.

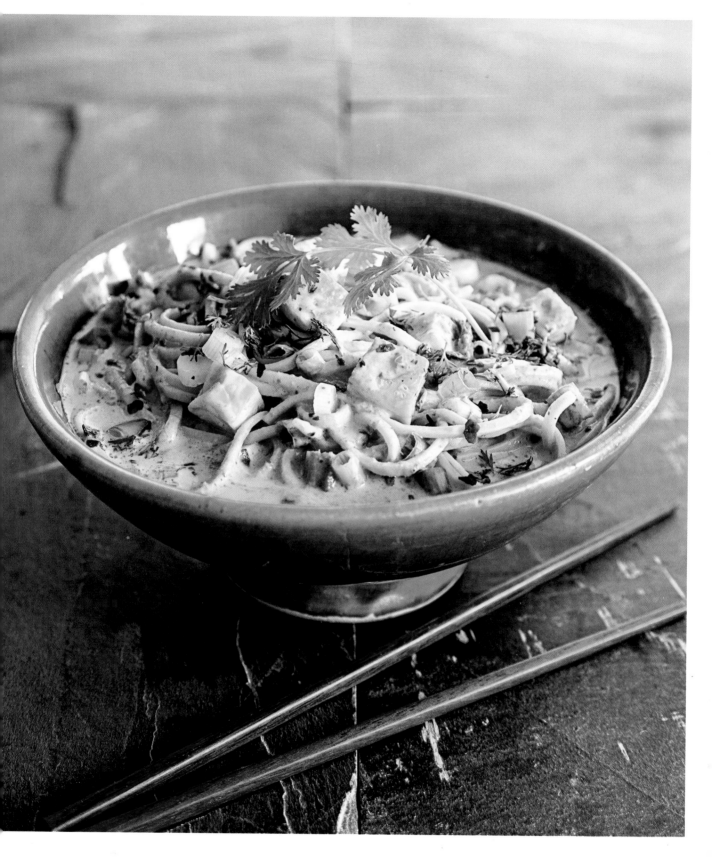

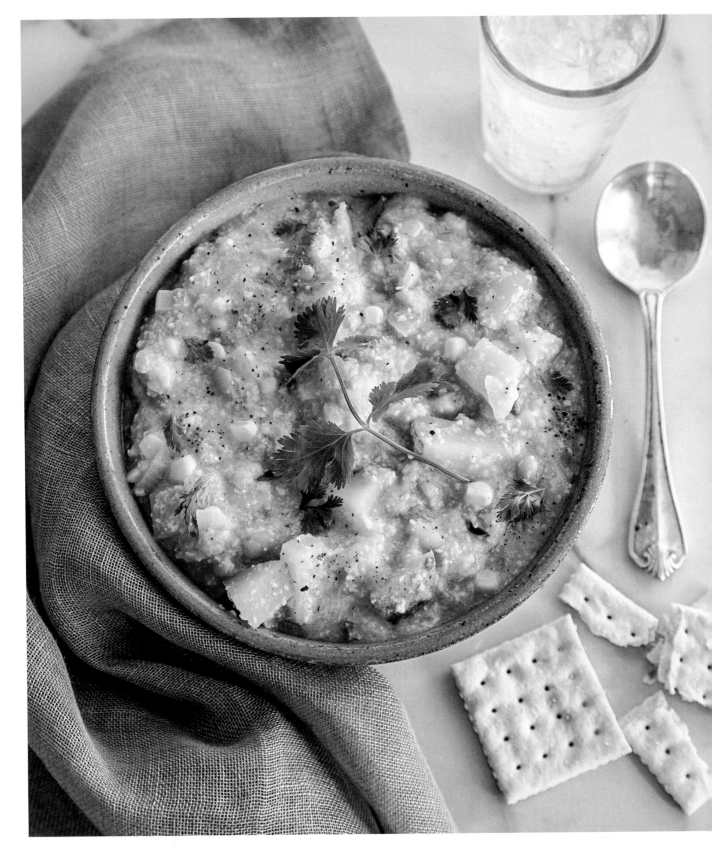

VEGAN CLAM CHOWDER

When I was a kid (Jess here), I used to love clam chowder. Then I realized that it included clams, and I sort of clammed up. I've never been a fan of meat, and seafood can really gross me out sometimes. We created this recipe for all of the non-clam, clam chowder lovers out there. We added white beans, soy milk and cashews to balance out the starch with a little protein. We also made sure to get our veggies in and snuck 1 cup (124 g) of chopped cauliflower into the mix. The variations of this recipe are basically endless. So after making it once, feel free to play around with it by adding or taking out anything you'd like.

Gluten-free (if using gluten-free vegetable broth and excluding the saltines or using gluten-free ones) / Vegan

Serves: 2
Per Serving (Calculation includes 2 saltines per serving) / **Calories:** 484 / **Carbohydrates:** 69 g / **Protein:** 17 g / **Fat:** 18 g

- ½ cup (69 g) raw, unsalted cashews
- 1 cup (237 ml) water
- 1 ear fresh white corn
- 1 tsp vegetable oil
- ½ yellow onion, diced
- 1 stalk celery, diced
- ½ yellow bell pepper, diced
- 4 cloves garlic, diced
- 1 small potato, chopped
- 1 cup (237 ml) vegetable broth
- 1 tbsp (8 g) garlic powder
- 2 sprigs fresh thyme
- 1 tbsp (4 g) dried oregano
- 1 cup (124 g) chopped cauliflower
- ½ cup (120 ml) soy milk
- ½ cup (90 g) white beans
- 1 tsp cornstarch
- Salt and pepper to taste
- ¼ cup (15 g) chopped cilantro, for garnish
- 4 saltine crackers (optional)

Soak the cashews in the water for 30 minutes. Meanwhile, cut the kernels off the ear of corn. The easiest way to do this is to cut the cob in half, then stand one end in the middle of a plate. Hold the corncob securely and cut the kernels off the cob all the way around. Repeat with the other corncob half.

Heat the vegetable oil in a pot over medium heat, then add the diced onion, celery and bell pepper. Let that cook for about 4 minutes, stirring occasionally until the vegetables begin to soften and then add the garlic. Cook until fragrant, about 2 to 4 minutes more. Now add the chopped potato, corn and vegetable broth. Add garlic powder, thyme and oregano and stir to combine. Cover with a lid and cook for 10 minutes, stirring occasionally until the potatoes are tender. While that's cooking, place the cashews with soaking water, chopped cauliflower and soy milk in a high-speed blender. Blend for 1 to 2 minutes, or until fully puréed.

When the soup has started to thicken, add the white beans and then mix in the cornstarch and finally the cashew-cauliflower purée. Lower the heat to a simmer and cook for 5 to 10 minutes longer, until the chowder is thick and creamy (yet slightly chunky). Add salt and pepper to taste. Keep in mind that this makes two huge portions. Store any leftovers in an airtight container in the fridge or freezer. Garnish with the chopped cilantro and serve each bowl with 2 saltines, if desired.

SPICY THAI TOFU TACOS WITH PEANUT SAUCE

A lot of our patients think tacos are off limits when it comes to eating healthy, but it's quite the opposite. If you include lots of veggies in your tacos, bake the shells, choose lean protein and lay off the extra cream and cheese, tacos are almost a superfood. For example, in this recipe, we focus on baking the shells to a crispy perfection, instead of frying. This recipe also provides about 1½ cups (105 g) of fiber-rich vegetables like cabbage and carrots. And you're definitely getting your dose of protein with the crispy tofu and peanut sauce. Nutrition aside, this recipe is absolutely delicious, so let's get started.

Gluten-free (if using gluten-free soy sauce) / Vegan

Serves: 2

Per Serving / Calories: 496 / **Carbohydrates:** 53 g / **Protein:** 20 g / **Fat:** 24 g

TACOS

- ½ (16-oz [454-g]) block extra-firm tofu
- 1 tsp vegetable oil
- 6 corn tortillas
- Pinch of paprika
- 4 scallions
- 1 small handful of cilantro, plus more for garnish
- ⅔ carrot, grated
- 2 tsp (4 g) grated fresh ginger
- 1 cup (70 g) shredded purple cabbage
- Sriracha sauce to taste

DRESSING

- Juice of ½ lime
- 1 tsp rice vinegar
- 1 tsp toasted sesame oil
- Pinch of salt
- ½ recipe Peanut Sauce (page 141)

For the tacos, remove the tofu from the package and wrap it in a clean towel. Use half of the block for this recipe and save the remaining half for later by submerging it in water (in an airtight container) and storing it in the refrigerator for 3 to 5 days. Place the towel-wrapped tofu in a glass pan, then put something heavy on top. The idea is to press all of the water out of the tofu for up to 4 hours. When the tofu is drained, cut it into small cubes (about ½ x ½-inch [1.3 x 1.3-cm]).

Preheat the oven to 375°F (190°C). Coat a baking sheet with the oil.

Spread the cubed tofu pieces on the prepared baking sheet and bake for 30 minutes, flipping the tofu with a spatula halfway through so it cooks evenly. Keep the oven on.

Cook the tortillas in the oven using our crunchy, no-fry baking method. Drape each tortilla over one or two bars of the oven rack and bake until crispy, 4 to 8 minutes depending on your oven. You can spray the tortillas with a little cooking spray first if you want to add extra crunch. Sprinkle with a pinch of paprika for flavor.

Chop the scallions and cilantro, then add them to a bowl. Add the grated carrot next, then the ginger and purple cabbage.

For the dressing, combine the fresh lime juice, vinegar and sesame oil in a small bowl. Mix well, then drizzle it over the veggies and toss to coat. Top the veggie mixture off with a pinch of salt.

When the tofu is heated, mix it with the peanut sauce. Then divide the tofu among your crispy taco shells. Divide the vegetable medley among the tacos as well. Top with a small handful of cilantro for garnish and Sriracha if you're in the mood for a little spice. Enjoy!

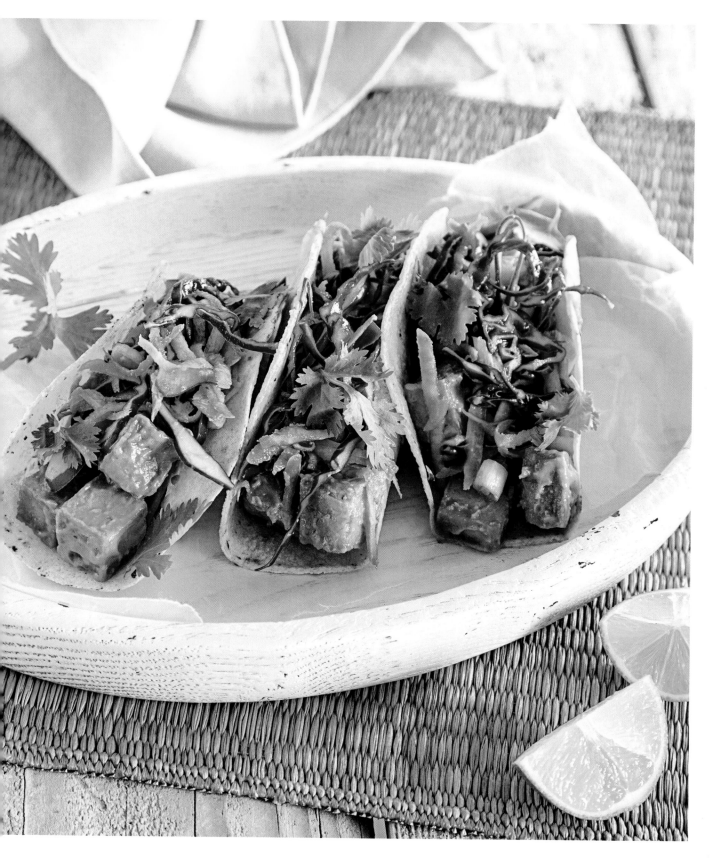

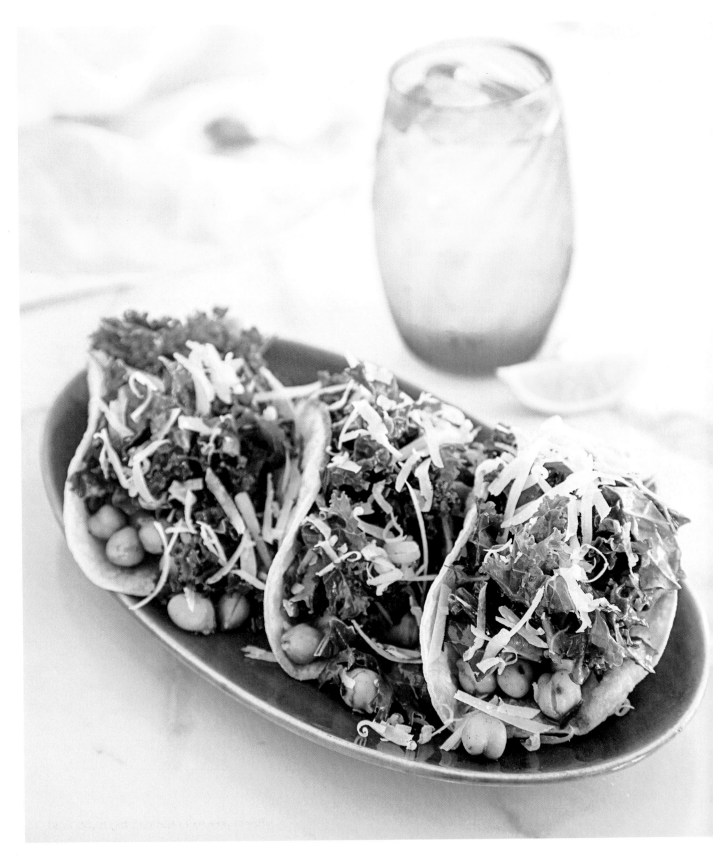

CHICKPEA KALE TACOS WITH PARMESAN CHEESE

Nobody loves tacos more than we do. Okay, maybe everybody loves tacos as much as we do. And can you blame the world? Tacos hit our four food heaven pillars: they're super delicious, easy as all heck to make, very healthy if you add the right ingredients and best of all, cheap. In fact, when we have dinner parties, tacos are one of our go-to grubs, because you can feed a village for the price of a venti Caramel Macchiato at Starbucks®.

Gluten-free / 30 minutes or less

Serves: 1 / **Calories:** 424 / **Carbohydrates:** 66 g / **Protein:** 15 g / **Fat:** 12 g

- 3 small corn tortillas
- A pinch of paprika
- ½ cup (82 g) cooked chickpeas
- A pinch of salt
- ¼ tsp chili powder
- ¼ tsp crushed red pepper flakes
- 2 cups (32 g) finely chopped kale
- ½ tsp olive oil
- Juice of ¼ lemon
- 1 tsp grated Parmesan cheese

Cook the tortillas in the oven using our crunchy no-fry baking method (see the Spicy Thai Tofu Tacos with Peanut Sauce recipe on page 150).

Place the chickpeas in a bowl and add a pinch of salt, the chili powder and red pepper flakes. Stir to mix then set aside.

Place the chopped kale in a bowl. Add the olive oil and a pinch of salt and massage the leaves for about 30 seconds, until the kale softens. Sprinkle with the lemon juice.

Divide the chickpeas between the three tacos and top with the kale. Finish it all off with the grated Parmesan.

LENTIL FALAFEL WITH CUCUMBER DILL YOGURT SAUCE

This easy recipe is a twist on falafel, which is traditionally made with chickpeas; we use lentils as a base instead. Per ounce (28 g), lentils have more fiber (16 g) and protein (18 g) than most other beans, and they are ridiculously simple to cook because they don't require any soaking. You can also do what we did and buy precooked lentils to save even more time. The kicker in this recipe is the yogurt sauce, which is healthier than a traditional white sauce (we use 2% Greek yogurt) but doesn't lack in flavor.

Serves: 2
Per Serving / **Calories:** 521 / **Carbohydrates:** 86 g / **Protein:** 37 g / **Fat:** 4 g

FALAFEL

· ¾ cup (144 g) dried lentils or 2 cups (396 g) cooked lentils

· ¼ red onion, finely chopped

· 1 small handful of cilantro

· 2 cloves garlic

· ½ tsp chili powder

· ½ tsp ground cumin

· ½ tsp garlic powder

· 2 tsp (5 g) 100% whole-wheat flour

YOGURT SAUCE

· 1 cup (245 g) 2% Greek yogurt

· ¼ cup (33 g) diced cucumber

· 1 tsp chopped dill

· Juice of ½ lemon

· ½ clove garlic

· Salt and pepper to taste

TO SERVE

· Two 100% whole-wheat pita breads

· 6 tomato slices

· ½ cup (10 g) arugula

Preheat the oven to 400°F (204°C).

For the falafel, if your lentils aren't already cooked, boil them in a pot filled with water for about 20 minutes, or until tender. Allow the lentils to cool, then drain the water. In a food processor, combine the cooked lentils, red onion, cilantro, garlic cloves, chili powder, cumin and garlic powder. Pulse until crumbly, but not sticky. Make sure that you don't go overboard by puréeing the mixture. Slowly sprinkle in the flour and pulse to evenly combine throughout the mixture.

Use your hands to form the lentil mash into four balls and place on a nonstick baking tray. Slightly flatten them so the shape is between a falafel ball and a burger. Bake for 15 minutes on one side, then flip over with a spatula and bake for an additional 15 minutes.

While the falafel is in the oven, make the yogurt sauce. Pulse the yogurt, cucumber, dill, lemon juice, garlic and salt and pepper to taste in a food processor until smooth.

Cut each of the pita breads in half around the outer edges so you have four round "slices" of pita. If you prefer your pita bread toasted, toast in the oven for a few minutes. Top one slice with half of the yogurt sauce, three slices of tomato, two pieces of falafel and arugula. Then form your sandwich by adding the second slice of pita on top. Alternatively, you can stuff the ingredients into the open pita halves as pictured. Repeat to form a second sandwich. Enjoy!

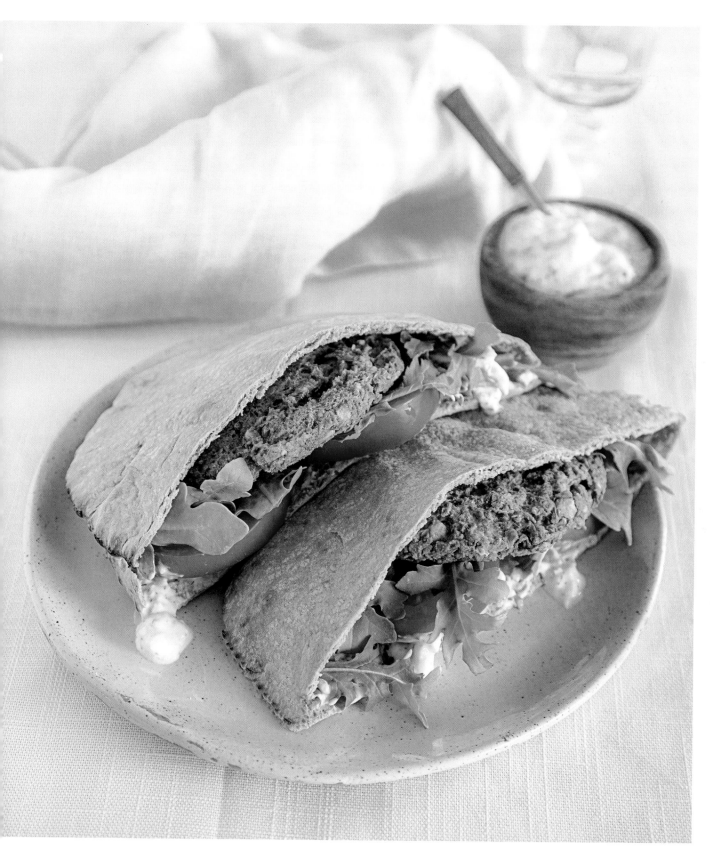

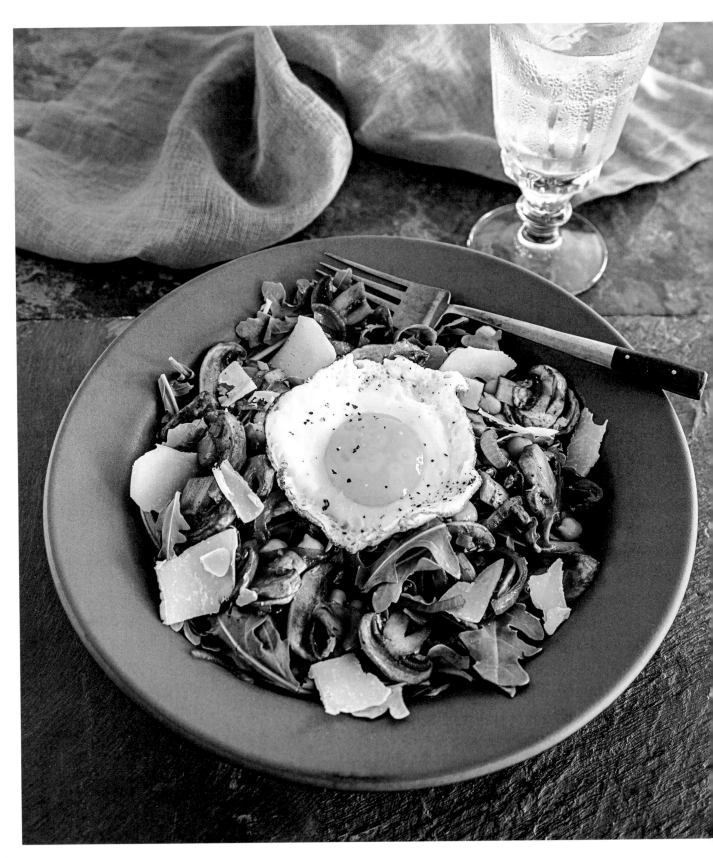

MUSHROOM ARUGULA SALAD

Arugula offers a distinct, peppery flavor, which makes it the perfect ingredient for a robust and aromatic salad. A cruciferous vegetable, arugula is a rich source of glucosinolates, which have been suggested to have protective effects against different types of cancers. The sharp flavor of Parmesan cheese goes perfectly with this herbaceous leafy green. Add the protein-rich egg and chickpeas and you have yourself a light, nourishing meal.

Gluten-free / 30 minutes or less

Serves: 1 / **Calories:** 423 / **Carbohydrates:** 32 g / **Protein:** 25 g / **Fat:** 21 g

- 2 cups (40 g) arugula
- 1 tsp olive oil
- ¼ onion, sliced
- 1½ cups (108 g) sliced button mushrooms
- 1 tbsp (10 ml) balsamic vinegar
- ½ cup (82 g) cooked chickpeas
- 1 oz (28 g) shaved Parmesan cheese
- 1 egg
- Salt and pepper to taste

Place the arugula in a bowl and set aside. In a pan, heat the olive oil and add the sliced onions. Cook for 2 minutes over medium heat, stirring occasionally, until the onions are fragrant, and then add the mushrooms and balsamic vinegar. Cook for 3 to 4 minutes with the lid on, until the mushrooms are a golden color. Remove from the heat and let cool. Add to the bowl with the arugula, then add the chickpeas and shaved Parmesan.

Prepare the egg your favorite way. We went with an egg over easy, because the runny yolk pairs deliciously with the arugula and mushrooms. However, you can also enjoy this salad with a boiled or poached egg. Top the salad with your prepared egg, season with salt and pepper and dig in.

FILLING WHITE BEAN KALE SALAD WITH GARLIC LEMON DRESSING

Fact: We used to find raw kale salads very intimidating. Let's be honest—kale is kind of rough and all that chewing can really tire out your jaw. But we're going to let you in on a little secret. You can make any kale salad absolutely delicious and easy to eat if you do this one simple step: massage it. That's right—kale needs to be massaged in a bit of oil to break down some of those fibers and make it more palatable. You also need to add salt (a little goes a long way) in order to remove the sometimes bitter flavor. Do these two things and you'll end up with a magical raw kale salad every time.

Gluten-free / Vegan / 30 minutes or less

Serves: 1 / **Calories:** 470 / **Carbohydrates:** 51 g / **Protein:** 20 g / **Fat:** 20 g

SALAD

- **4 cups (64 g) finely chopped kale**
- **1 tsp olive oil**
- **A pinch of freshly ground salt**
- **½ small avocado**
- **½ carrot, peeled**
- **1 tsp chopped onion**
- **½ cup (90 g) cooked Great Northern beans or any white bean**

GARLIC LEMON DRESSING

- **1 clove garlic (if you're a garlic lover, use 2)**
- **1 tsp olive oil**
- **Juice of 1 lemon**
- **Salt and pepper to taste**

For the salad, we'll start by giving the kale a good ol' massage. First, place the chopped kale in a bowl. Add olive oil and a pinch of fresh cracked salt. Massage the leaves for about 30 seconds, or until the kale softens. Next, chop the avocado into cubes and slice the carrot into thin rounds. Add the avocado, carrot, onion and beans to the kale and toss to combine.

For the dressing, dice the garlic, then add to a bowl with the olive oil and lemon juice. Season with salt and pepper to taste. Pour onto the salad and mix well. Enjoy!

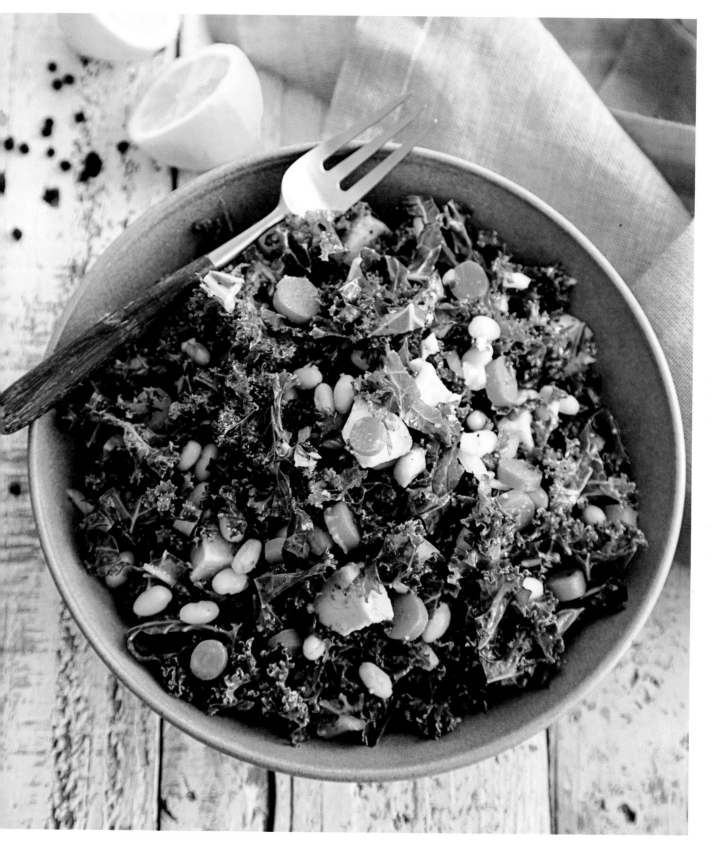

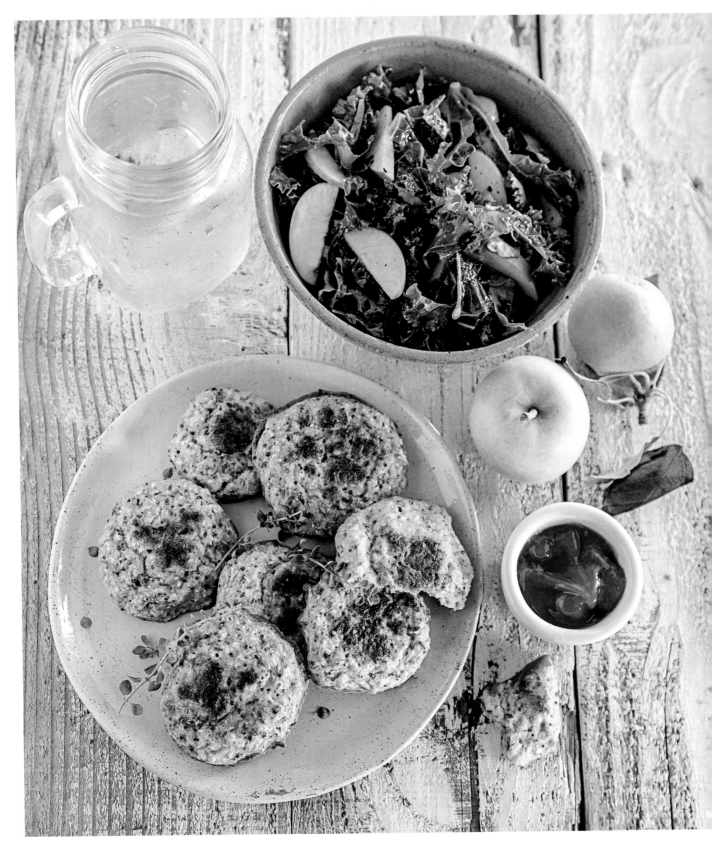

CAULIFLOWER AND BROCCOLI "CHICKEN" NUGGETS

I haven't had an actual chicken nugget since the first grade (Jess here). I didn't like them then, and I probably wouldn't like them now. But these cauliflower and broccoli "chicken" nuggets get a gold star in my book. This has to be the easiest way to add 2 cups (215 g) of veggies to a dish without a second thought. We chose cauliflower and broccoli because they are great for baking, and as cruciferous veggies, they are top of the line as far as nutrition is concerned. Cruciferous vegetables are some of the highest sources of vitamin A carotenoids, vitamin C, folic acid and fiber. Just beware that for some, cruciferous veggies can cause bloating and gas. If this happens to you, consider popping a digestive enzyme before this meal.

Serves: 2

Per Serving / **Calories:** 385 / **Carbohydrates:** 57 g / **Protein:** 18 g / **Fat:** 12.5 g

CAULIFLOWER AND BROCCOLI "CHICKEN" NUGGETS

- 1 cup (124 g) chopped cauliflower
- 1 cup (91 g) chopped broccoli
- 1 clove garlic
- 2 eggs
- ¼ tsp chopped fresh thyme
- ¼ tsp chopped fresh oregano
- A pinch of salt and pepper
- ⅓ cup plus 1 tablespoon (50 g) 100% whole-wheat flour
- 2 tbsp (30 g) ketchup

KALE APPLE SIDE SALAD

- 6 cups (100 g) chopped kale
- 1 tsp olive oil
- A pinch of salt
- 1 apple, sliced
- Juice of 1 lemon
- 2 tbsp (16 g) chopped pecans

Preheat the oven to 375°F (190°C). Oil a baking sheet.

For the nuggets, combine the cauliflower, broccoli and garlic clove in a food processor and pulse until the mixture resembles a crumbly cauliflower rice. Remove it from the food processor and transfer it to a large bowl. Add the eggs, thyme, oregano and a pinch of salt and pepper, then stir to mix well. Gradually add the flour and stir until all the ingredients are fully combined.

Oil your hands, to prevent the mixture from sticking to them, then form the mixture into 8 to 10 "nugget" balls and place them on the prepared baking sheet. Bake for 25 to 30 minutes, or until the outside is crispy and the inside is moist—just like a chicken nugget. Flip halfway through for even cooking.

While the nuggets are baking, make the side salad to pair with this dish. Place the kale in a bowl, add the olive oil and a pinch of salt, and massage the kale until softened, about 30 seconds. Add the sliced apple and drizzle with the lemon juice. Sprinkle the pecans on top and enjoy the salad alongside the nuggets. Use ketchup for dipping.

SPIRALIZED ZUCCHINI PESTO PASTA

We kept seeing spiralizer recipes posted all over Instagram, but didn't want to believe the hype. How could one device completely revolutionize the way we cook? It sounded too good to be true. And then we got one. In short, it changed our lives. Love pasta? No problem. Substitute a cup of spiralized zucchini noodles to cut the calories in half. If you have trouble getting 3 cups (680 g) of vegetables into your daily life, this could be your answer. Our advice: If you don't have a spiralizer, get one now (although this recipe can easily be made without one!).

Vegan

Serves: 2
Per Serving / **Calories:** 618 / **Carbohydrates:** 66 g / **Protein:** 15 g / **Fat:** 32 g

PASTA

- 4 oz (113 g) dried whole-wheat spaghetti
- 2 medium zucchini
- 10 cherry tomatoes
- 2 tsp (10 ml) vegetable oil
- 12 pitted black olives
- 12 pieces sun-dried tomato

ARUGULA PESTO*

- 2 cups (40 g) arugula
- ½ cup (80 ml) olive oil
- ¼ cup (60 ml) water
- ¼ cup (35 g) almonds
- 2 cloves garlic
- Salt and pepper to taste

For the pasta, cook the spaghetti according to package directions. Drain and place in a bowl.

While the noodles are cooking, make the pesto. Place the arugula, olive oil, water, almonds and garlic in a food processor and pulse until a paste forms. Season to taste with salt and pepper.

Spiralize the zucchini using a spiralizer. If you don't have a spiralizer, cut the zucchini using a vegetable peeler to form long ribbons.

Slice the cherry tomatoes in half and set aside.

Heat the vegetable oil in a pan over medium heat. Add the spiralized zucchini and tomatoes to the pan, cover with a lid and cook until fragrant but still firm, 4 to 5 minutes; stir occasionally. Remove from the heat, then add the cooked whole-wheat pasta and toss to combine. Top with ⅓ cup (84 g) of the pesto and sprinkle with the olives and sun-dried tomatoes.

Note
This recipe makes about 1 cup (252 g) of pesto. You will use ⅓ cup (83 g) of pesto in this recipe and save the rest for other recipes as part of the sample week-1 meal plan. You can store the pesto in an airtight container in the refrigerator for up to 1 week.

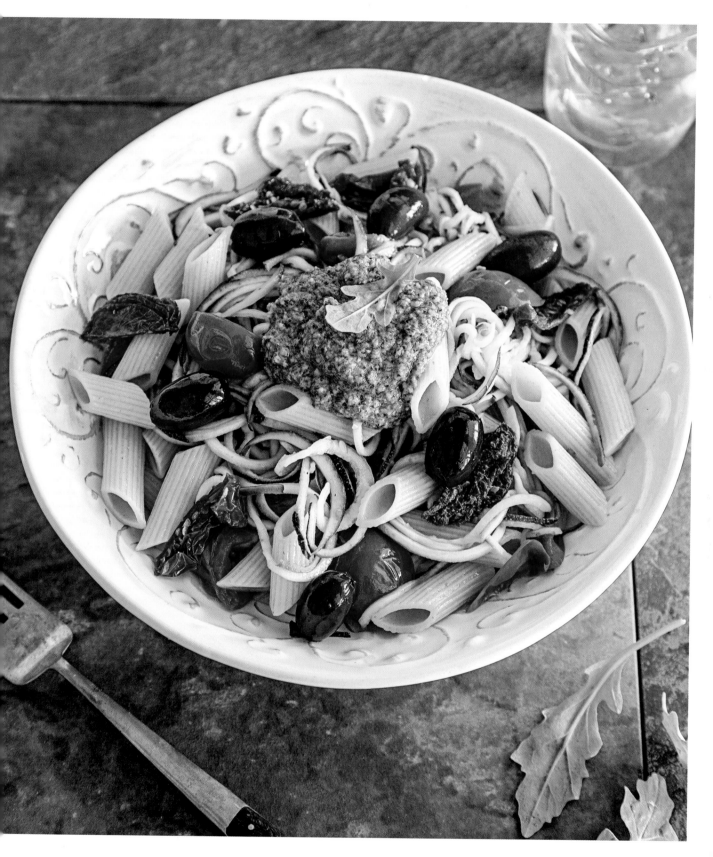

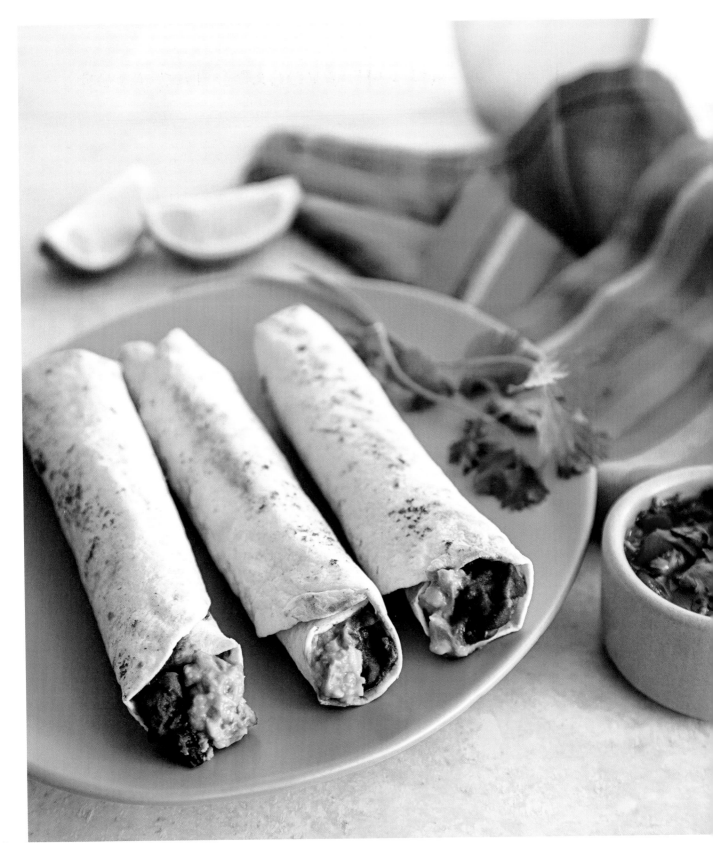

OIL-FREE BLACK BEAN AND AVOCADO TAQUITOS

Black beans are the best. For starters, beans are one of the world's best sources of fiber. A ½-cup (93-g) serving, of black beans in particular, is packed with almost 8 grams of fiber, which is more than 30 percent of your daily needs (note: at minimum, women should try to eat 28 grams of fiber per day while men should aim for 35 grams). Fiber is great at supporting the body's natural detoxification process, helping to strengthen the colon and keep you regular in the process. Black beans are also a good source of protein, containing 9 grams per every ½-cup (93-g) serving. Enjoy this healthy spin on a traditional Mexican dish for dinner any night of the week.

30 minutes or less

Serves: 1 / **Calories:** 591 / **Carbohydrates:** 87 g / **Protein:** 24 g / **Fat:** 19 g

TAQUITOS

- ½ cup (93 g) cooked black beans
- ½ avocado
- ½ tsp ground cumin, divided
- ½ tsp chili powder, divided
- 3 small flour tortillas

SALSA

- 1 tomato
- ½ shallot
- Juice of 1 lime
- 1 clove garlic
- 1 tsp chopped cilantro
- Salt and pepper to taste

- ¼ cup (61 g) 2% Greek yogurt

Preheat the oven to 425°F (218°C). Have a baking sheet handy.

For the taquitos, mash the black beans and avocado in two separate bowls. Mix half of each of the cumin and chili powder into the black bean mash.

Next, spread the tortillas on a baking sheet. Bake until hot, about 2 minutes, then transfer to a plate, hot side down. Add an inch-wide (2.5-cm) line of avocado and black beans across the diameter of each tortilla. If you have kids, they will have fun with this part.

Roll the filled tortillas up into a tightly wrapped cigar shape. Top each taquito with the remaining half of the cumin and chili powder. Coat the baking sheet with cooking spray. Place the stuffed taquitos on the baking sheet and bake until crispy, 15 to 20 minutes.

While the taquitos are cooking, make the super easy salsa. Place the tomato, shallot, lime juice, garlic and cilantro in a food processor and pulse a few times until chopped but still chunky. If you don't have a food processor, you can chop manually and mix. Add salt and pepper to taste.

Enjoy the taquitos with the salsa and Greek yogurt as your "sour cream."

CREAMY SPINACH ARTICHOKE QUESADILLAS

These creamy quesadillas are complemented by the sweet undertones of red onion sautéed with brown sugar. This dish is incredibly easy to make and provides more than 30 percent of your daily fiber needs. Fiber is essential for maintaining gut health and helping manage blood sugar. It also helps with weight management and provides protection against heart disease.

Gluten-free / 30 minutes or less

Serves: 1 / **Calories:** 418 / **Carbohydrates:** 60 g / **Protein:** 14 g / **Fat:** 14 g

- 1 tsp olive oil
- Pinch of brown sugar
- ¼ small red onion, chopped
- 3 cloves garlic, minced
- ½ cup (84 g) canned artichoke hearts, drained, rinsed and sliced
- 2 cups (60 g) raw spinach
- ½ tbsp (7.5 g) cream cheese
- 4 corn tortillas
- 2 tbsp (14 g) shredded pepper Jack cheese
- Salt and cayenne pepper to taste

In a pan, heat the olive oil and brown sugar for 30 seconds over medium-low heat, or until the brown sugar starts to bubble. Then add the chopped onion and garlic. Sauté for 1 minute over medium heat. Add the sliced artichokes to the pan and cook for 3 minutes, or until lightly browned, stirring occasionally. Add the spinach and cream cheese. Place the cover on the pan and cook for 2 minutes. Remove the cover, stir well to distribute the cream cheese, and cook for another 2 minutes with the lid off. Remove from the heat and set aside.

Place 2 corn tortillas on a plate and divide the spinach artichoke mixture between them. Top with the shredded cheese and sprinkle with salt and cayenne pepper to taste. Top each with the remaining corn tortillas and cook on a grill press for 8 minutes, or until the tortillas have browned and the cheese has melted. You can also do this on the stove. Simply place the layered tortillas in a pan and cook for 3 minutes on each side, until the tortillas have browned and the cheese has melted. Slice each quesadilla into 4 wedges. Enjoy!

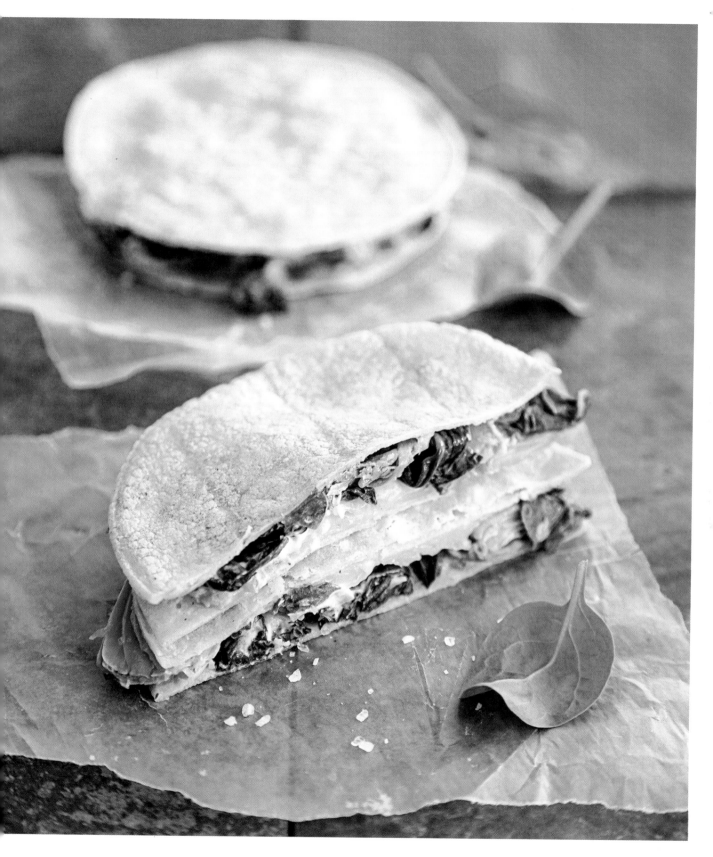

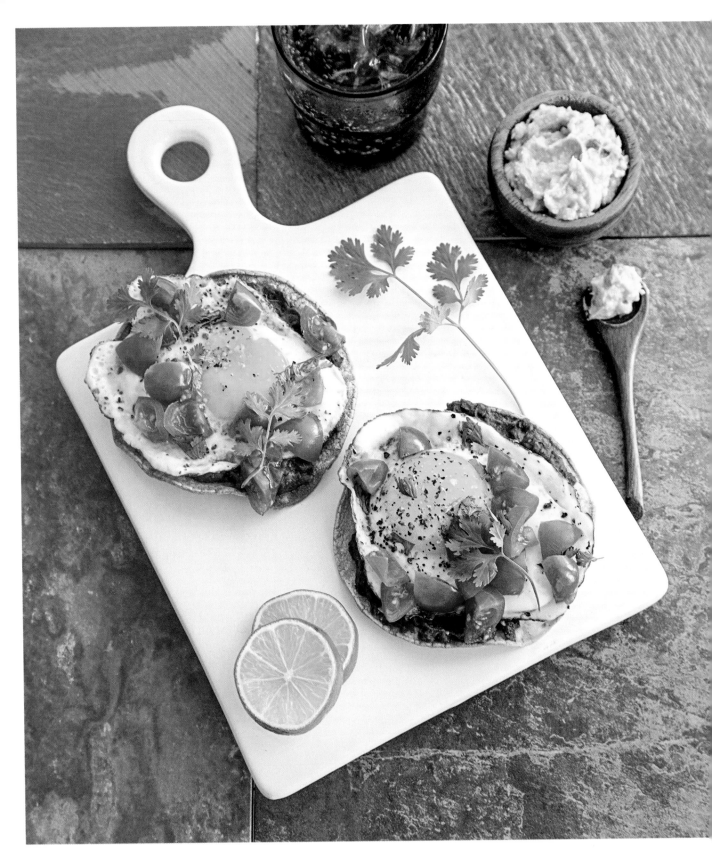

QUICK AND EASY HUEVOS RANCHEROS TOSTADAS

Ask any New Yorker what they've got planned at 11 a.m. on a Sunday morning and the answer is always "brunch." Friends, drinks, food—I mean really, what more is there to life? When we go a-brunchin', one of our favorite dishes to order is the classic huevos rancheros. It's vegetarian-friendly, filling and tastes delicioso. We made this traditional breakfast dish into a hearty dinner by turning the huevos rancheros into tostadas. We absolutely love eggs because they help balance out the carbohydrates in the meal by offering a punch of perfect protein. Also, instead of frying the beans, we got the same effect by mashing them, which makes this dish even healthier.

Gluten-free / 30 minutes or less

Serves: 1 / **Calories:** 477 / **Carbohydrates:** 47 g / **Protein:** 24 g / **Fat:** 24 g

- 2 small corn tortillas
- ⅛ jalapeño pepper, seeded
- ⅓ small avocado
- Juice of ½ lime
- ½ cup (93 g) cooked black beans
- ¼ tsp chili powder
- ¼ tsp ground cumin
- ¼ tsp onion powder
- ¼ tsp garlic powder
- Salt and pepper to taste
- 1 tsp vegetable oil
- 2 eggs
- A small handful of cilantro, chopped
- 5 cherry tomatoes, sliced

Preheat the oven to 375°F (190°C).

Cook the tortillas in the oven using our crunchy no-fry baking method. Simply place the flat tortillas on the baking rack and bake until crispy, 4 to 8 minutes, depending on your oven.

Dice the jalapeño and add it to a bowl with the avocado and lime juice. Mash together until it is a mostly creamy but slightly chunky dressing.

Add the black beans, chili powder, cumin, onion powder and garlic powder to a bowl. Mash until the mixture resembles refried beans. Add salt and pepper to taste. Set aside.

Heat the vegetable oil in a pan over medium-high heat. Wash the eggs and then crack them over the pan. Lower the heat immediately and cook for about 6 minutes, or until the yolk barely starts to set. If you want the yolk runny, stop now, but if you like it firmer, cook for a few more minutes. Sprinkle with a tad of salt and pepper.

Spread the black bean mash on the tostadas, place 1 egg over each, top with the cilantro and tomatoes and drizzle with the sauce. Enjoy!

GARLIC ARTICHOKE PITA PIZZA

Pita pizzas win for effortless cooking. You literally throw your favorite ingredients onto a pita, pop it into the oven and 15 minutes later you have yourself a full-blown dinner. For this recipe, we create a garlicky ricotta and vegetable sauté that will serve as the topping for the pizza. Ricotta cheese is a great source of protein and comes loaded with calcium and selenium. It adds a light creaminess to this recipe that is both satisfying and delectable.

30 minutes or less

Serves: 1 / **Calories:** 421 / **Carbohydrates:** 51 g / **Protein:** 16 g / **Fat:** 19 g

- 1 tbsp (15 ml) olive oil
- 4 cloves garlic, minced
- ½ cup (84 g) canned artichoke hearts, drained, rinsed and sliced
- ¼ cup (22 g) sliced Brussels sprouts
- 1 tbsp (16 g) light ricotta cheese
- One 100% whole-wheat pita
- ¼ cup (61 g) tomato sauce
- 2 tbsp (14 g) shredded mozzarella cheese
- Salt and black pepper to taste

Preheat the oven to 400°F (204°C). Line a baking sheet with parchment paper.

Heat the olive oil in a pan over medium heat, add the minced garlic and sauté for 2 minutes. Add the artichokes and Brussels sprouts to the pan and sauté for 4 minutes longer, stirring occasionally. Turn off the heat, add ricotta to the pan and mix in well with the sautéed vegetables. Set aside.

Place the pita on the prepared baking sheet and spread the tomato sauce on top. Top with the sautéed vegetable ricotta mix, and sprinkle the shredded mozzarella on top evenly. Bake for 15 minutes or until the cheese has melted and the pita edges are crisp. Season with salt and black pepper to taste.

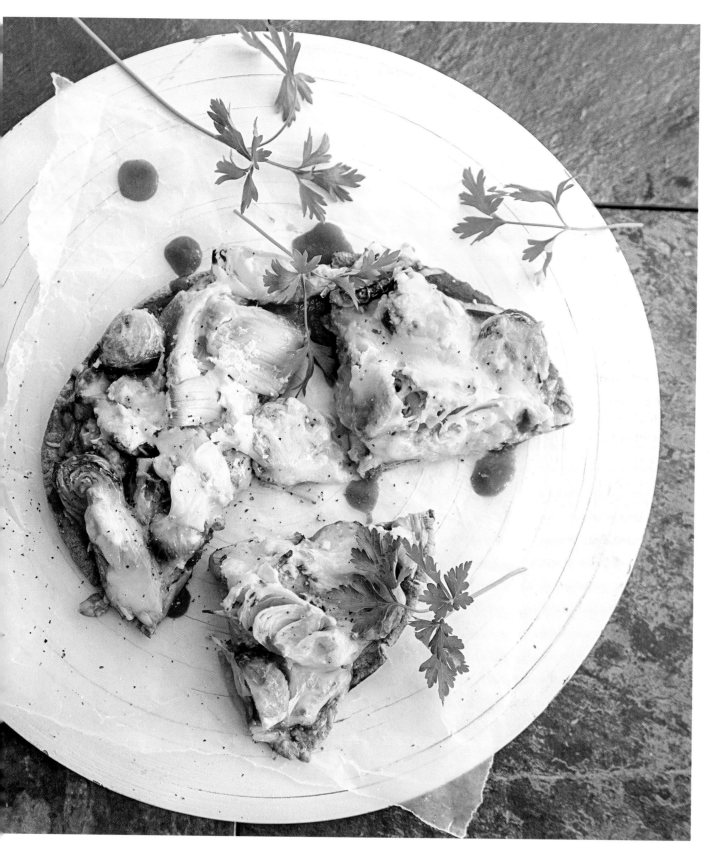

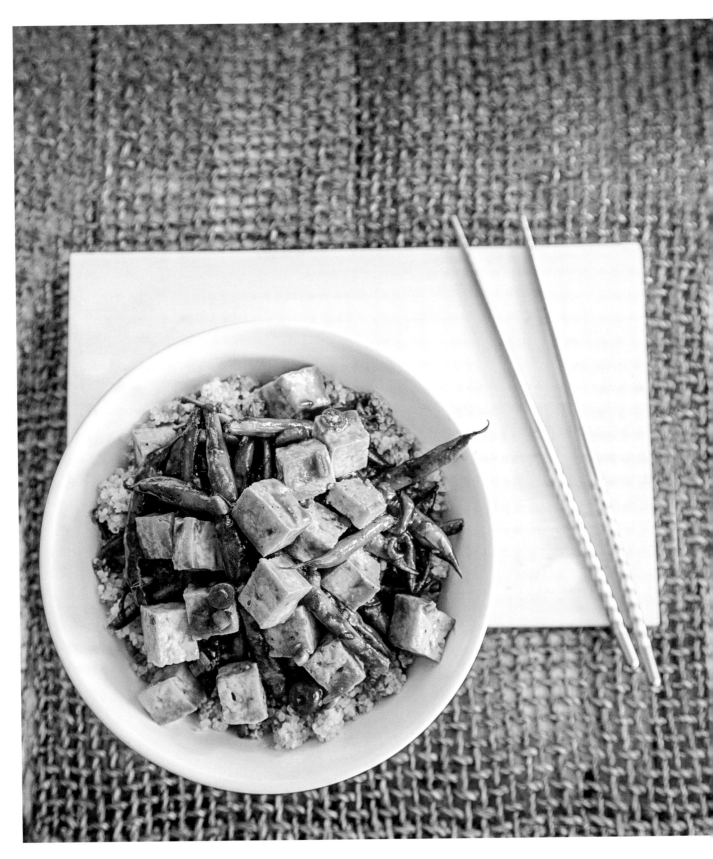

CRISPY BLACK PEPPER TOFU WITH GREEN BEANS

One of our favorite dishes to order at a Chinese restaurant is black pepper tofu. It's so rich, and creamy, and spicy, and crunchy—the perfect combination for a satisfying dish. We wanted to create a healthier version of black pepper tofu by using minimal (mostly whole) ingredients and baking the tofu instead of frying. We also serve over quinoa instead of white rice, because quinoa is one of the rare plant-based foods that's a complete protein (in addition to buckwheat and soy).

Gluten-free (if using gluten-free soy sauce) / Vegan

Serves: 2
Per Serving / Calories: 561 / **Carbohydrates:** 51 g / **Protein:** 30 g / **Fat:** 27 g

- 1 (16-oz [454-g]) block extra-firm tofu
- 3 tsp (30 ml) vegetable oil, divided
- 1½ cups (355 ml) water
- ½ cup (92 g) uncooked quinoa
- Salt to taste
- 2 tsp (5 g) cornstarch
- 4 tsp (20 ml) soy sauce
- 1 tsp black pepper
- 1 tsp diced fresh ginger
- 4 tsp (8 g) chopped scallion
- ½ cup (118 ml) water
- 2 cups (200 g) sliced green beans

Remove the tofu from the package and wrap it in a clean towel. Place it in a glass pan, then put something heavy on top. The idea is to press all of the water out of the tofu for up to 4 hours. When the tofu is drained, cut it into small cubes (about ½ x ½-inch [1.3 x 1.3-cm]).

Preheat the oven to 375°F (190°C). Coat a baking sheet with 1 teaspoon of the vegetable oil.

Spread the cubed tofu on the prepared baking sheet and bake for 30 minutes, flipping the tofu with a spatula halfway through. If you are eating this recipe as part of the sample week-1 reboot, use half of the tofu for this recipe and store the remainder in an airtight container in the refrigerator for future recipes. The tofu will remain fresh for up to 1 week.

In a small pot, bring the water to a boil over high heat, and then add the quinoa. Lower the heat to a simmer, cover with a lid and cook for 15 to 17 minutes. When the quinoa is soft and fluffy, add salt to taste and allow it to cool.

Combine the remaining 2 teaspoons (10 ml) of vegetable oil, the cornstarch, soy sauce, pepper, ginger and scallion in a bowl. Mix well, then set aside.

Add the water to a pan over medium heat, then add the green beans. Cover and let the green beans steam for 3 minutes, or until bright green (be careful not to overcook, these should still be crispy). If water remains in the pan after the green beans are done cooking, drain it.

Add the tofu and black pepper sauce to the same pan with the drained, cooked green beans. Stir to combine, then cook over medium heat for about 5 minutes. One of our tricks for knowing when things are done is the aroma. We promise that you'll start to smell all of the garlicky goodness once it's done cooking. Serve over a bed of quinoa and add salt to taste.

CAPRESE GRILLED CHEESE

There are an infinite number of reasons why the grilled cheese sandwich is a beloved staple in so many households. It's an incredibly easy meal to whip up, and the variations are endless. For this recipe, we'll be doing an Italian-inspired rendition, with mozzarella, tomatoes and basil. The sweetness of the basil really brings out the flavors of the tomato and mozzarella. In less than 10 minutes, you'll have a crispy bite of simplicity and perfection.

30 minutes or less

Serves: 1 / **Calories:** 411 / **Carbohydrates:** 47 g / **Protein:** 22 g / **Fat:** 17 g

- 2 slices 100% whole-grain bread
- 2 oz (56 g) mozzarella cheese, sliced into rounds
- 2 tomato slices
- 2 fresh basil leaves, chopped
- 1 tsp olive oil
- Salt and pepper to taste

Layer one slice of bread with the mozzarella cheese, tomatoes and fresh basil. Drizzle the olive oil on top. Add salt and pepper to taste, and top with the other slice of bread. Place it in a grill press and cook for 7 to 8 minutes, or until the cheese has melted and the bread has reached the desired crispness. If you don't have a grill press, you can cook it in a skillet over medium heat for 5 minutes on each side.

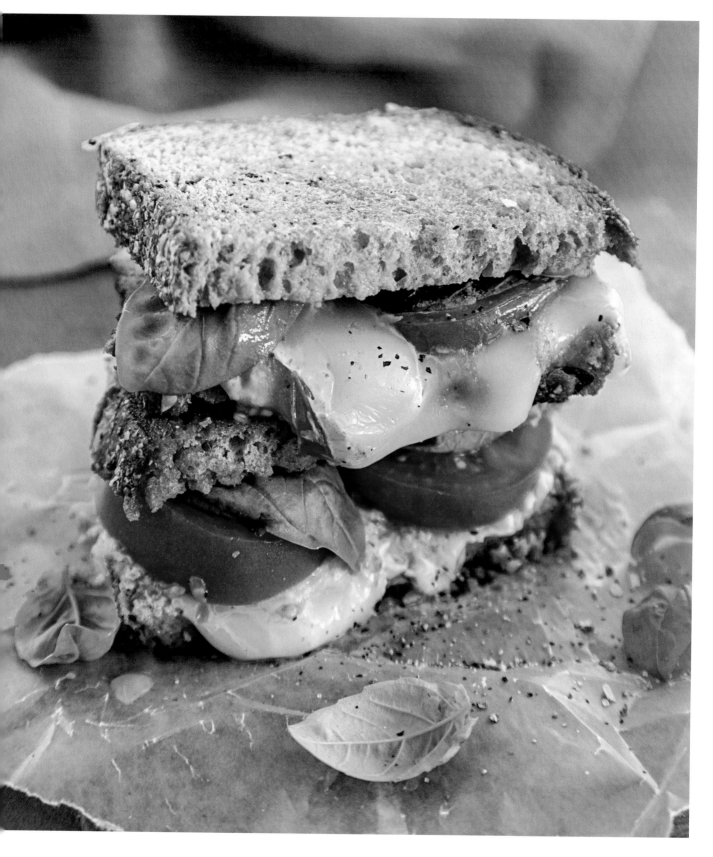

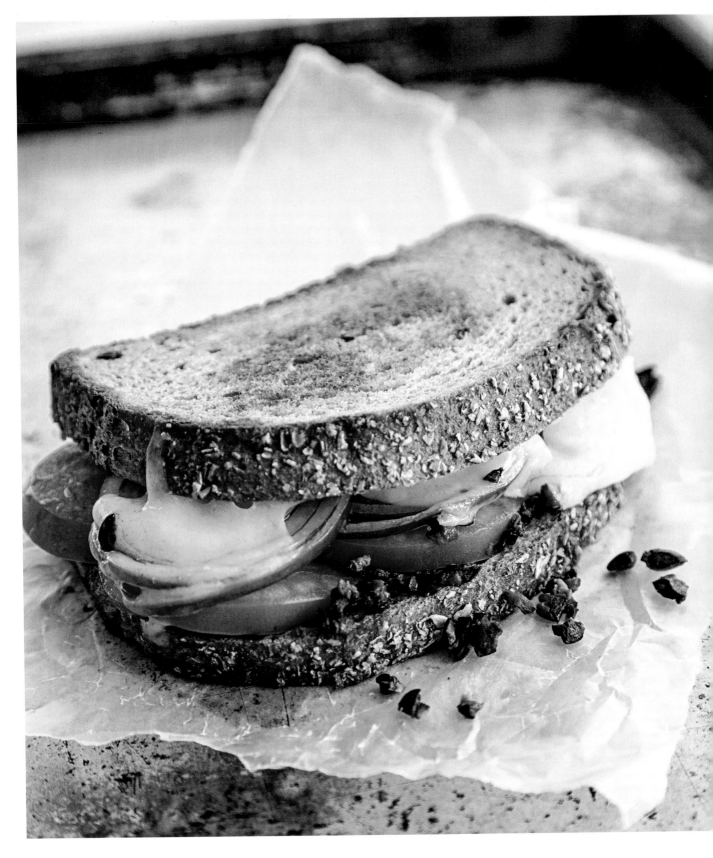

BLACK OLIVE GRILLED CHEESE

Black olives are a great addition to this sandwich because they provide a pop of acidic flavor that pairs brilliantly with melted cheese. Olives have anti-inflammatory and antioxidant properties, and provide heart-protective benefits thanks to their monounsaturated fat content. When using olives in recipes, it's best to minimize or completely avoid using additional salt, as olives are usually cured in salt.

30 minutes or less

Serves: 1 / **Calories:** 449 / **Carbohydrates:** 50 g / **Protein:** 21 g / **Fat:** 20 g

- 6 small pitted black olives
- 2 slices 100% whole-grain bread
- 3 tomato slices
- 3 red onion slices
- 2 oz (56 g) mozzarella, sliced into rounds
- 1 tsp olive oil

In a bowl, mash the black olives into a paste using a large spoon or a pestle. Spread the olive paste onto one slice of bread, and then pile on the tomato, onion and mozzarella cheese. Drizzle the olive oil on top, and then cover with the other slice of bread. Place it in a grill press and cook for 7 to 8 minutes, or until the cheese has melted and the bread has reached the desired crispness. If you don't have a grill press, you can cook it in a skillet over medium heat for 5 minutes on each side.

SPICY CHIPOTLE LENTIL TACOS

Lentils are an absolute nutrition powerhouse because they are jam-packed with both fiber and protein. In this taco recipe, the lentils resemble cooked ground beef or taco meat, which adds a fun twist. The kicker here is our vegan chipotle sauce, which (heads up!) is pretty spicy.

Gluten-free / Vegan

Serves: 1 / **Calories:** 631 / **Carbohydrates:** 89 g / **Protein:** 24 g / **Fat:** 23 g

TACOS

- ¾ cup (149 g) cooked black lentils or ¼ cup (48 g) dried lentils
- ½ tsp vegetable oil
- 1 tsp chopped onion
- 2 cloves garlic, minced
- 1 tsp chili powder
- 1 tsp paprika
- 1 tsp ground cumin
- 1 tsp garlic powder
- 1 tsp onion powder
- 1 tsp water (as needed)
- Salt and pepper to taste
- 2 scallions
- 7 cherry tomatoes
- 3 corn tortillas

CHIPOTLE SAUCE

- ¼ small avocado
- 1 chipotle pepper in adobo sauce
- 2 tsp (6 g) raw cashews, chopped
- ⅓ cup (80 ml) water
- Juice of ¼ lemon
- 1 tsp vegetable oil
- Salt and pepper to taste

For the tacos, if your lentils aren't cooked, boil them in a pot filled with water for about 20 minutes, or until tender. Let cool, then drain the water.

Heat the vegetable oil in a pan over medium heat. Add the onion and garlic and cook for 2 to 3 minutes, stirring frequently. Add the chili powder, paprika, cumin, garlic powder and onion powder and cook for 5 minutes longer. Add the cooked lentils and stir to combine. If the lentils begin to dry out, add the water as needed. The mixture should resemble moist, cooked ground beef. Add salt and pepper to taste.

Chop the scallions and cherry tomatoes and set aside.

Preheat the oven to 375°F (190°C). Drape each tortilla over one or two bars of the oven rack and bake until crispy, 4 to 8 minutes.

For the chipotle sauce, combine the avocado, chipotle pepper, cashews, water, lemon juice and vegetable oil in either a blender or a food processor and process until creamy. Add salt and pepper to taste.

Divide the cooked lentils among the tacos. Drizzle about 1 teaspoon of the chipotle sauce over each taco, then top with the scallions and cherry tomatoes.

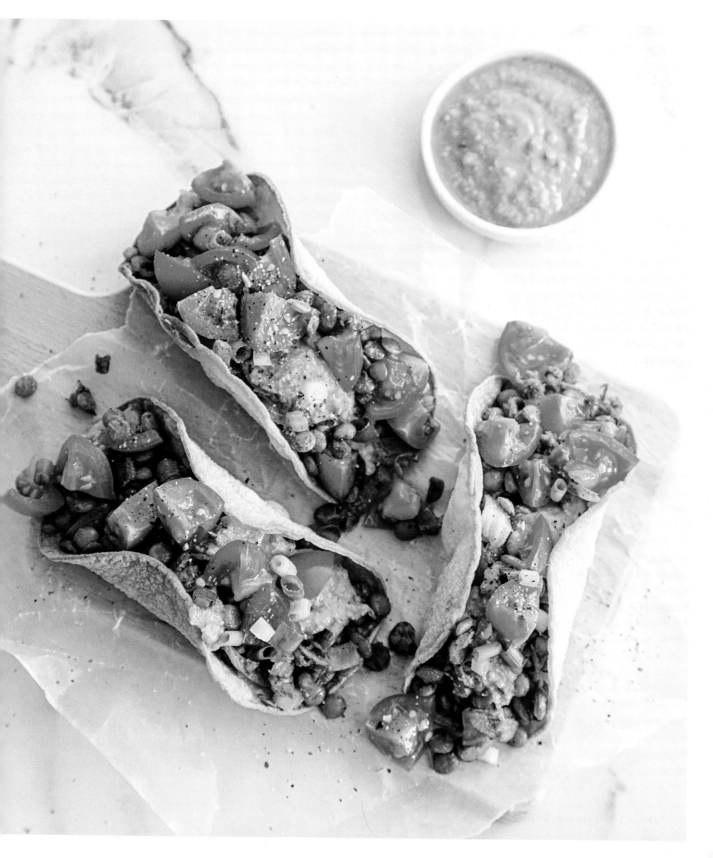

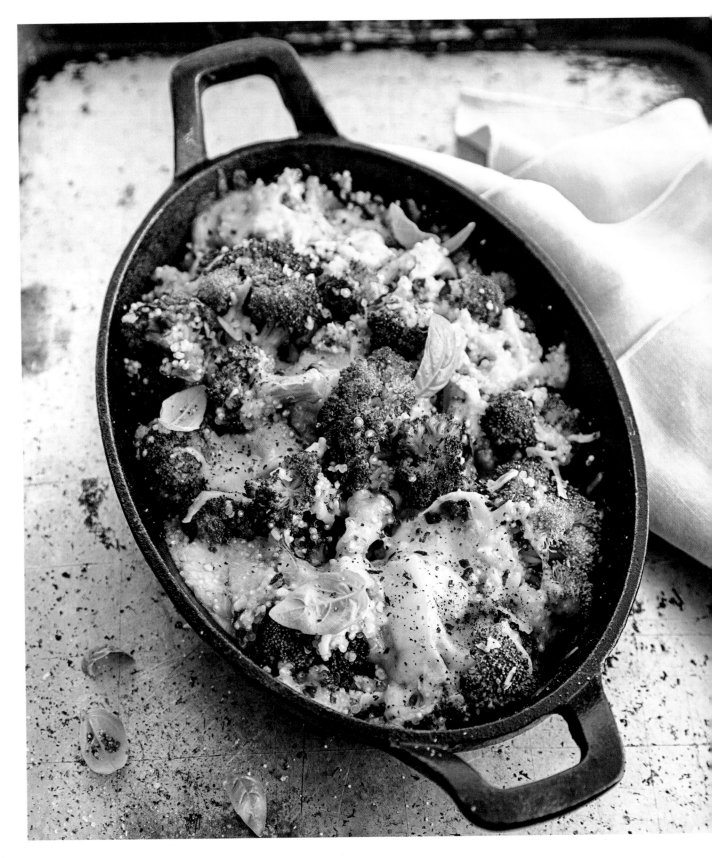

CHEESY GARLIC BROCCOLI QUINOA CASSEROLE

We use quinoa a lot throughout this book. That's because it's a nutritional powerhouse. It's one of the few grains that is also a complete protein, delivering all of the essential amino acids (or protein building blocks). We promise this recipe is just as flavorful as it is healthy. Crushed red pepper flakes provide a little heat.

Gluten-free (if using gluten-free vegetable broth)

Serves: 2

Per Serving / Calories: 573 / **Carbohydrates:** 70 g / **Protein:** 29 g / **Fat:** 19 g

- 2 tsp (6 g) minced garlic
- ⅓ cup (8 g) basil
- 2 tsp (10 ml) water
- 1 tsp olive oil
- 2 cups (182 g) broccoli florets
- 1 cup (170 g) uncooked quinoa
- 2 cups (473 ml) vegetable broth
- ¼ cup (25 g) grated Parmesan cheese
- ½ cup (57 g) part-skim mozzarella cheese
- ¼ tsp crushed red pepper flakes

Preheat the oven to 400°F (204°C). Oil an 8 x 8-inch (20.5 x 20.5-cm) baking dish.

In a food processor, combine the garlic, basil, water and olive oil and pulse to blend. Steam the broccoli in the microwave for 2 to 3 minutes, or until it turns bright green. If you don't have a microwave, place the broccoli in a pan and add 2 tablespoons (30 ml) of water. Cook for 3 minutes, or until bright green.

Meanwhile, combine the quinoa and vegetable broth in a pot, cover and bring to a boil over high heat. Boil for about 5 minutes and then stir. Drain the quinoa and add it, along with the slightly cooked broccoli and the garlic basil mixture, to the prepared baking dish. Stir to combine, then bake for 15 minutes.

Remove the baking dish from the oven and stir again. Sprinkle it with the Parmesan cheese, then the mozzarella, coating it evenly. Place the baking dish back in the oven and cook for an additional 20 minutes, stirring halfway through. Remove it from the oven and stir in the red pepper flakes. If you are only eating half of this casserole now, you can save the other half for another meal later; store it in a covered container in the refrigerator for up to 5 days.

MANGU WITH BARBECUE TEMPEH

Simply put, mangu is mashed plantains. The dish is a national favorite in the Dominican Republic and is typically enjoyed for breakfast with fried cheese, eggs and salami. It goes without saying that we had to remix things a bit to create a more veg-friendly version. This mangu is topped with a sweet and savory barbecue tempeh, an excellent source of plant-based protein that provides iron, calcium, magnesium and other essential minerals.

Gluten-free (if using gluten-free tempeh and soy sauce)

Serves: 1 / **Calories:** 584 / **Carbohydrates:** 75 g / **Protein:** 22 g / **Fat:** 23 g

MARINATED TEMPEH

- 3.5 oz (99 g) tempeh
- 1 tbsp (17 g) tomato paste
- ¼ tsp garlic powder
- ½ tsp maple syrup
- ½ tsp apple cider vinegar
- ¼ tsp soy sauce
- 1 tbsp (15 ml) water
- 1 tsp olive oil

MANGU

- 1 medium green plantain
- 1 tsp garlic powder
- 2 tsp (10 g) unsalted butter
- Salt and black pepper to taste

TOPPING

- ¼ medium onion, sliced
- 1 tsp balsamic vinegar

For the marinated tempeh, cut the tempeh in half lengthwise and place it in a bowl. In another bowl, whisk together the tomato paste, garlic powder, maple syrup, apple cider vinegar, soy sauce and water. Drizzle the sauce onto the tempeh, turn to coat and let it marinate for at least 20 minutes.

For the mangu, peel the plantain and chop it into 4 or 5 chunks. Bring a medium pot of water to a boil over high heat and add the plantain. Lower the heat to medium-high and cook the plantain for 35 to 40 minutes, or until soft and tender. Drain out most of the water from the pot, leaving about 3 to 4 tablespoons (45 to 60 ml) behind for mashing. Using a pestle or the bottom of a cup, mash the plantains well with the remaining water, add the garlic powder and butter, and continue mashing until a smooth consistency has been reached. Scoop the mangu into a serving bowl and season it with salt and black pepper to taste.

To cook the tempeh, heat the olive oil in a skillet over medium heat, add the tempeh slices and cook them for 3 minutes on each side. Place them over the mangu. To keep the dish warm while you prepare the onion topping, cover the bowl with a lid.

For the topping, add the onion slices to the same pan the tempeh was cooked in. Add the balsamic vinegar, stir to coat and cook for 2 to 3 minutes over medium heat.

Top the mangu and tempeh with the onions, and you're ready for a mouthwatering meal!

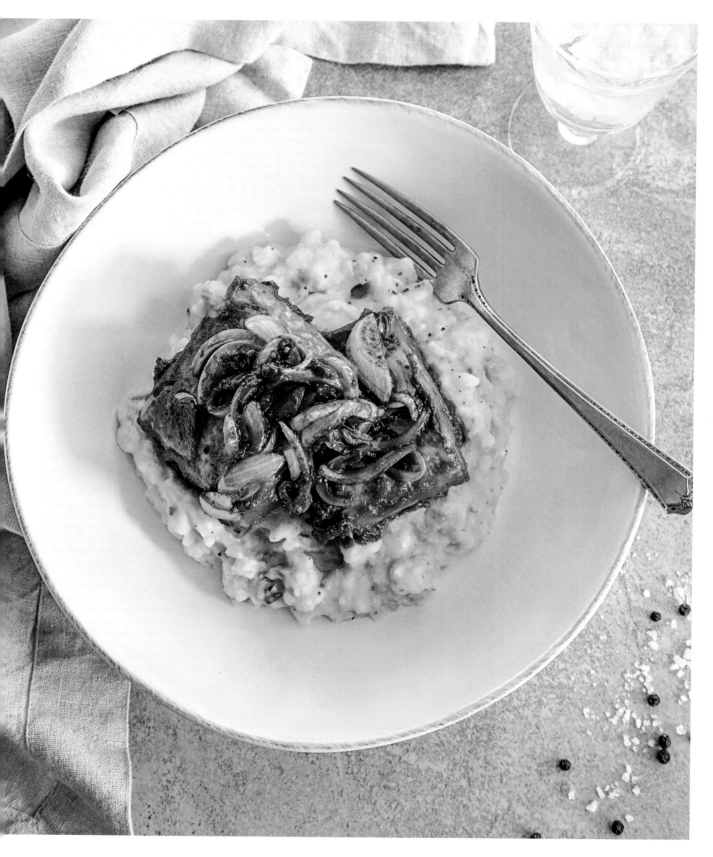

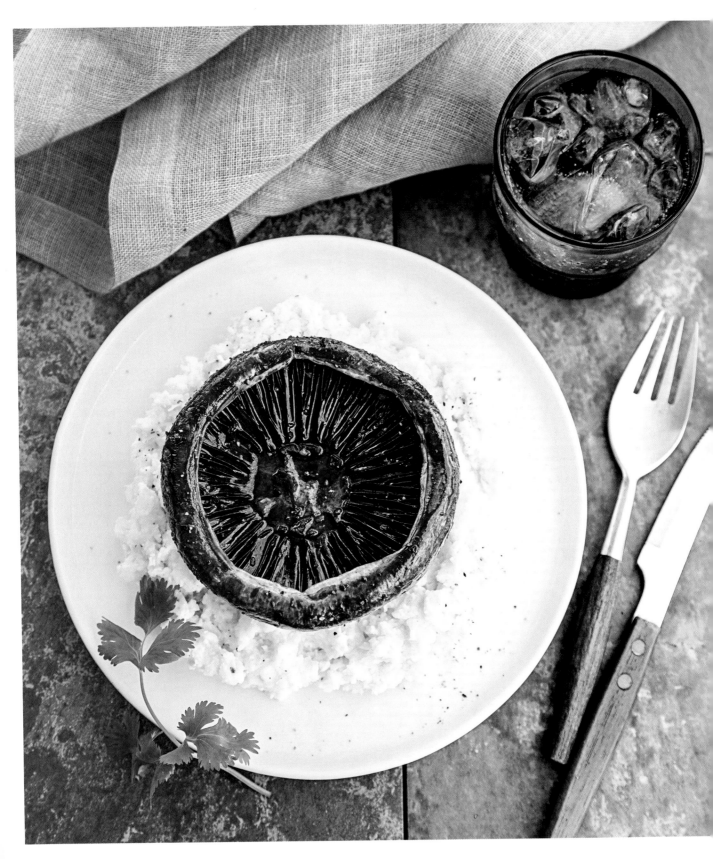

CREAMY CAULIFLOWER MASHED POTATOES WITH SOY-GLAZED PORTOBELLO

Creamy and garlicky cauliflower mashed potatoes? Life can't get any better than this. Having cauliflower in mashed potatoes is one of the many ingenious ways you can incorporate more vegetables (and nutrition) into meals. Our soy-glazed portobello mushroom complements this dish beautifully and provides an additional dose of fiber, B vitamins, selenium, phosphorus and potassium.

Gluten-free (if using gluten-free soy sauce) / 30 minutes or less

Serves: 1 / **Calories:** 405 / **Carbohydrates:** 40 g / **Protein:** 9 g / **Fat:** 14 g

- 1 small potato
- 1 portobello mushroom
- 1 tsp soy sauce
- 1½ tsp (7.5 ml) olive oil, divided
- 1 tsp rice vinegar
- ¼ tsp ground black pepper
- 1½ cups (186 g) cauliflower florets
- 2 cloves garlic, minced
- ½ tbsp (7 g) cream cheese
- Salt to taste

In a pot of water, boil the potato for 15 to 20 minutes, or until tender.

While the potato is cooking, remove the stem from the portobello and place it in a bowl with the gills facing up. Add the soy sauce, 1 teaspoon of olive oil, rice vinegar and ground black pepper and let it marinate for 10 to 15 minutes.

Pulse the cauliflower florets in a food processor until a fine, grainy texture has been reached.

Heat ½ teaspoon of olive oil in a skillet over medium heat and add the minced garlic. Sauté for 1 minute, and then add the pulsed cauliflower. Sauté for 3 to 4 minutes, stirring occasionally, until the cauliflower is tender, then transfer it to a bowl. Add the cooked potato and cream cheese, and using a large spoon or pestle, mash all of the ingredients together until creamy. Add salt to taste, and set aside.

Cook the portobello on a grill press for 5 minutes. Alternatively, cook the mushroom in a skillet over medium heat for 3 minutes on each side. Top the potato/cauliflower mash with this savory mushroom, and you're all set for a delicious meal!

EGGPLANT GYRO

This loaded eggplant gyro is a succulent alternative to the traditional meat gyro. The eggplant absorbs the wonderful flavors of the paprika and oregano, and once cooked, it makes a colorful and fragrant stuffing for your pita. Adding chickpeas and hummus to this dish is an excellent way to boost the fiber and protein content, and topping it with the cucumber and parsley makes for a refreshing finish!

Vegan / 30 minutes or less

Serves: 1 / **Calories:** 452 / **Carbohydrates:** 65 g / **Protein:** 15 g / **Fat:** 17 g

- 1½ cups (123 g) chopped eggplant
- 1 tsp dried oregano
- ½ tsp paprika
- 2 tsp (10 ml) olive oil
- Small pinch of salt
- One 100% whole-wheat pita bread
- 3 tbsp (46 g) hummus
- ¼ cup (33 g) chopped cucumber
- ¼ cup (45 g) chopped tomato
- 4–5 thinly sliced onion rounds
- 2 tbsp (21 g) cooked chickpeas
- 1 tbsp (4 g) fresh parsley
- Salt and black pepper to taste

Add the chopped eggplant to a bowl and add the oregano, paprika, olive oil and a light pinch of salt. Using a spoon or your hands, mix the eggplant with the spice mix so that all of the eggplant is coated. Heat a skillet over medium-low heat, add the eggplant, cover with a lid and cook for 8 to 10 minutes, mixing occasionally.

Heat the pita bread for 2 to 3 minutes in a pan on the stovetop, in the oven or in a grill press. Spread the hummus onto the pita bread, and once the eggplant is done, add that on as well. Then top with the cucumber, tomato, onion, chickpeas and fresh parsley. Season with salt and pepper to taste.

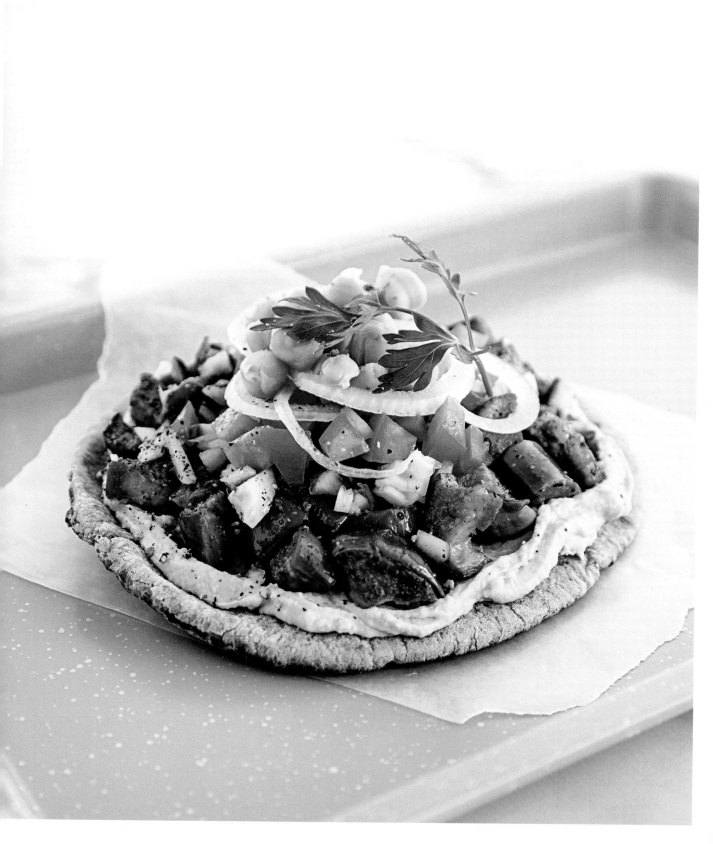

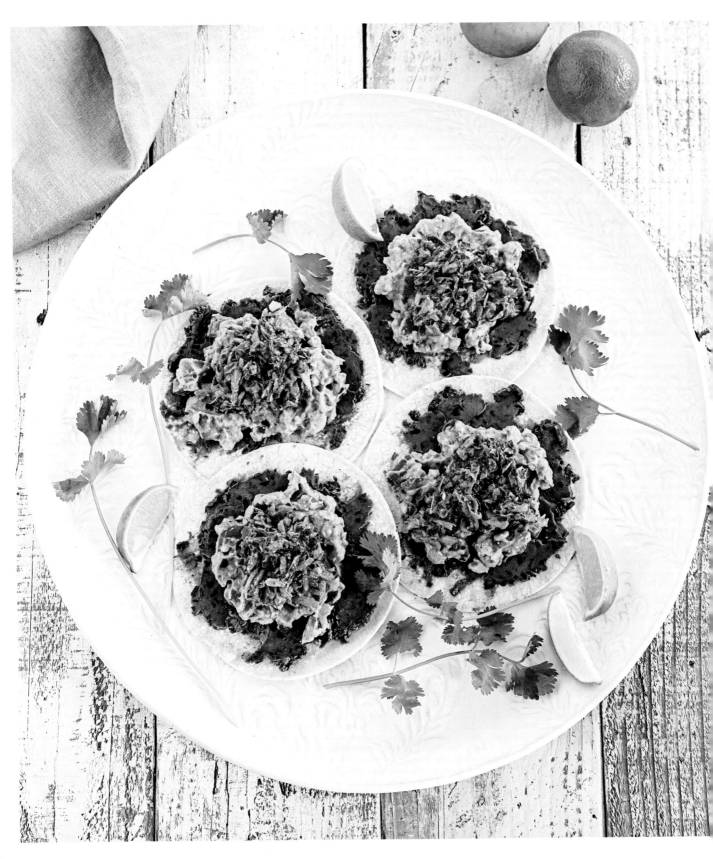

GUACAMOLE TACOS WITH RED CABBAGE SLAW

Avocados are hands-down one of our favorite foods. They are incredibly filling and provide an array of vitamins, minerals and other powerful nutrients. They help increase the absorption of fat-soluble vitamins A, D, E and K, and their creaminess works well in so many recipes. They are the main ingredient in these zesty tacos, which are stuffed with protein-rich black beans and topped with red cabbage slaw.

Gluten-free (if using gluten-free Dijon mustard) / Vegan / 30 minutes or less

Serves: 1 / **Calories:** 493 / **Carbohydrates:** 75 g / **Protein:** 11 g / **Fat:** 17 g

RED CABBAGE SLAW

- ½ cup (35 g) shredded red cabbage
- ¼ cup (32 g) shredded carrot
- 1½ tsp (20 ml) apple cider vinegar
- 1½ tsp (8 g) Dijon mustard

GUACAMOLE

- ½ Hass avocado
- ½ medium tomato, cubed
- ¼ red onion, chopped
- ⅓ jalapeño, seeded and chopped
- 1 tbsp (1 g) chopped cilantro
- Juice of ½ lime
- Salt to taste

BLACK BEANS

- ¼ cup (46 g) cooked black beans
- ½ tsp ground cumin
- Salt to taste
- 4 corn tortillas

For the slaw, combine the shredded red cabbage and carrot in a bowl. Add the apple cider vinegar and Dijon mustard and mix well. Set aside.

For the guacamole, combine the avocado, tomato, onion, jalapeño, cilantro and lime juice in another bowl. Using a fork or pestle, mash together, and then add salt to taste.

For the black beans, combine the beans, cumin and salt (to taste) in a third bowl. Mash together with a fork until the beans resemble a paste.

Heat the tortillas for 1 to 2 minutes on each side in a pan on the stove top or in a grill press. Place the tortillas on a plate and spread a thin layer of the black bean paste onto each. Then add the guacamole and top with the red cabbage slaw.

CHICKPEA TABBOULEH

Tabbouleh is a simple vegetarian dish that uses parsley as one of the main ingredients. Just 1 cup (60 g) of this aromatic herb covers more than 100 percent of your daily vitamin A and C needs! Since we'll be enjoying this as a meal, we added chickpeas for additional protein and calories.

Vegan / 30 minutes or less

Serves: 1 / **Calories:** 391 / **Carbohydrates:** 66 g / **Protein:** 11 g / **Fat:** 8 g

- ¾ cup (178 ml) water
- ¼ cup (35 g) cracked bulgur
- 1 cup (60 g) finely chopped parsley
- ½ cup (67 g) chopped cucumber
- ¼ medium onion, chopped
- ½ cup (90 g) cubed tomato
- 5 mint leaves, chopped
- ½ cup (82 g) cooked chickpeas
- ½ tbsp (7 ml) olive oil
- Juice of ½ lemon
- ¼ tsp black pepper
- Salt to taste

In a small pot, bring the water to a boil over high heat, add the bulgur, decrease the heat to medium-low, cover with a lid and cook for 15 minutes. Drain and let cool for 8 to 10 minutes.

Combine the parsley, cucumber, onion, tomato, mint and chickpeas in a bowl. Add the cooled bulgur, olive oil, lemon juice and black pepper, and stir to combine. Add salt to taste.

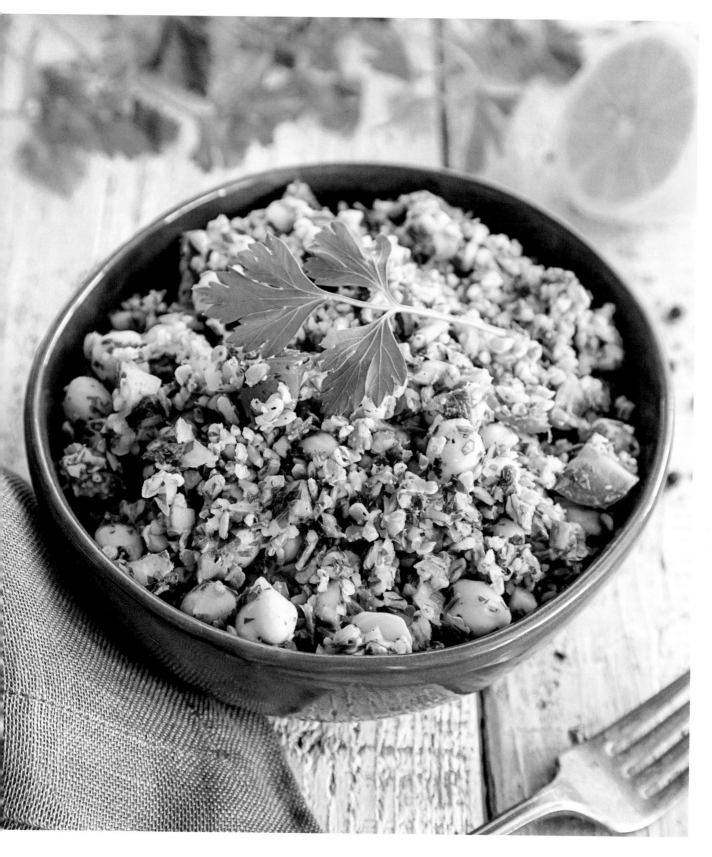

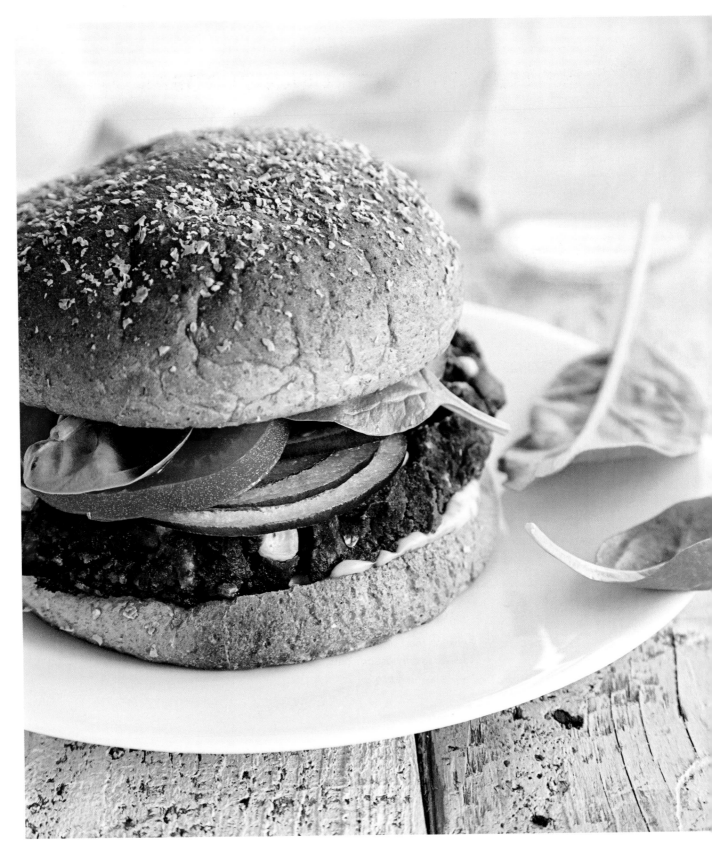

BUTTERNUT SQUASH BLACK BEAN BURGERS

Why purchase overprocessed veggie burgers when you can just make your own? These fiber-rich burgers are the official backup plan for days when you don't want to cook. You can make them in batches, freeze them, and when you get home, tired and not wanting to do much prep, simply thaw and cook! Note that to make oat flour, you simply process rolled oats in a blender or food processor until they reach a flour-like consistency.

Vegan

Serves: 2

Per Serving / **Calories:** 222 / **Carbohydrates:** 34 g / **Protein:** 7 g / **Fat:** 3 g

- ½ cup (70 g) peeled and cubed butternut squash
- ½ cup (93 g) cooked black beans
- ½ jalapeño, seeded and chopped
- 1 tsp tomato paste
- ½ tsp garlic powder
- ½ tsp ground cumin
- ½ tsp chili powder
- ½ cup (82 g) corn kernels
- ¼ cup (37 g) chopped red bell pepper
- ¼ cup (26 g) oat flour
- Salt to taste
- 4 slices 100% whole-grain toast or two 100% whole-grain buns

Preheat the oven to 400°F (204°C). Line a baking sheet with parchment paper.

Bring a pot of water to a boil over high heat, add the butternut squash, decrease the heat to maintain a simmer, cover with a lid and cook for 20 minutes, or until you can easily stick a fork through the squash. Remove it from the heat, drain the water and allow the squash to cool. Add the squash, black beans, jalapeño, tomato paste, garlic powder, cumin and chili powder to a food processor. Blend until you have a thick, consistent paste.

Scoop the paste into a bowl and add the corn and red bell pepper. With a spoon, mix the vegetables into the paste. Slowly add in the oat flour, mixing well with the other ingredients. Add salt to taste and place the bowl in the refrigerator for at least 30 minutes.

When cooled, remove the bowl from the refrigerator and, using a large spoon, scoop out half of the burger mix. Using your hands, form a round patty and set it on the prepared baking sheet. Repeat with the remaining mixture.

Bake for 15 minutes, and then flip the patties with a spatula and bake for another 15 minutes. Alternatively, you can cook these in a lightly oiled skillet or pan over low to medium heat for 5 minutes on each side, or until each side is crisp and browned.

Serve on toast or buns. Enjoy this with your favorite greens and/or toppings! If you're cooking just one patty, you can store the other one in the refrigerator for up to 1 week, or freeze for up to 1 month.

SNACK WISELY

Healthy snacking in between meals is a great way to curb your appetite until the next mealtime comes around. We created ten nourishing snack recipes that will provide you with energy in between meals. Snacks like our Spicy Dark Chocolate–Covered Almonds (page 196) and Chewy Cranberry Energy Balls (page 203) are easy to eat when you're on the go. Alternatively, you can enjoy our Guacamole with Baked Tortilla Chips (page 195) and Blackberry Jam Chia Pudding for those days when you have a little extra time. When snacking, be mindful and chew slowly to avoid overeating. Also be sure to stick to just one serving. The amount of snacks you have per day really depends on your appetite and nutrition goals. If you are interested in weight loss, we advise you to snack only when hungry. For those looking to boost your daily caloric intake, consider incorporating a tasty snack between each meal. If you want to maintain your weight but love to snack, eat smaller meals and add snacks in between. The way you set it up is entirely up to you!

BLACKBERRY JAM CHIA PUDDING

This pudding makes for a great yogurt alternative! It's super easy to whip up, and it can be customized with your favorite fruit and/or toppings. Chia seeds contribute a healthy dose of fiber, protein and omega-3s, and they can also be incorporated into smoothies, oatmeal, baked goods and more!

Gluten-free

Serves: 2
Per Serving / **Calories:** 186 / **Carbohydrates:** 22 g / **Protein:** 7 g / **Fat:** 8 g

- 1 cup (256 g) blackberries
- 1 cup (240 ml) unsweetened almond milk
- ½ tbsp (10 ml) honey
- ¼ cup (41 g) chia seeds

Add the blackberries, almond milk and honey to a blender. Blend until smooth, and then pour it into a jar or bowl. Slowly stir in the chia seeds until evenly dispersed. Refrigerate for at least 1 hour, or until firm. Divide between 2 bowls and enjoy. Feel free to top with your favorite nuts or seeds for an extra crunch!

GUACAMOLE WITH BAKED TORTILLA CHIPS

The secret to the perfect guacamole isn't in the avocados (yes, they are important)—it's the lime. For whatever reason, choosing lime over lemon adds the perfect tart citrus punch that takes any guacamole up several notches. We love pairing guac with these baked tortilla chips as the perfect snack that keeps us satiated for hours (thanks mostly to the healthy fats in the avocado). Avocados are the perfect cleansing food because of the monounsaturated fat content. Most people don't realize that eating healthy fats will actually help you absorb more of the fat-soluble vitamins in your diet—so don't be scared of them. Researchers have found that adding a side of avocado to salads, sweet potatoes, greens, carrots or tomato sauce increases carotenoid (a form of vitamin A) absorption from all of these foods.

Gluten-free / Vegan / 30 minutes or less

Serves: 1 / **Calories:** 169 / **Carbohydrates:** 23 g / **Protein:** 3 g / **Fat:** 8 g

- 1 small corn tortilla
- ½ roma tomato
- ⅓ small ripe avocado
- ½ clove garlic
- Juice of ½ lime
- 1 tsp chopped cilantro leaves
- Salt to taste

Preheat the oven to 350°F (177°C). Line a baking sheet with parchment paper.

Slice the tortilla in half, then slice those halves in half, and repeat the process one more time, until you have eight triangles. Spread on the prepared baking sheet and bake for about 5 minutes, or until crispy.

Add the tomato, avocado, garlic, lime juice, cilantro and salt (to taste) to a food processor and pulse until you get a chunky guac. Depending on your food processor, you may have to chop the avocado and tomato into a couple of large pieces before processing, so it pulses evenly. Enjoy the guacamole with the chips for the perfectly balanced snack.

SPICY DARK CHOCOLATE–COVERED ALMONDS

These almonds provide the perfect boost of energy for those of you who slowly drift away as the day progresses. Dark chocolate is rich in polyphenols, flavanols, catechins and other powerful antioxidants. Some studies have even shown that the flavanols in dark chocolate can improve circulation and may help with blood pressure control. Keep in mind that although nutritious, chocolate is a concentrated source of calories and fat. Stick to just 1 to 2 ounces (28 to 56 g) per day.

Gluten-free / Vegan

Serves: 8
Per Serving (11–12 almonds) **/ Calories:** 176 **/ Carbohydrates:** 8 g **/ Protein:** 5 g **/ Fat:** 14 g

- **1 cup (138 g) unsalted almonds**
- **1 (100-g) bar dark chocolate (70% cacao or more)**
- **Cayenne pepper and sea salt to taste**

Line a baking sheet with parchment paper.

Place the almonds in a bowl. Break the chocolate bar into 3 or 4 smaller pieces, and place in a small saucepan. Warm over low heat for about 3 minutes, stirring frequently with a spoon, until all the chocolate is melted. You can also melt the chocolate using the double boiler method. Simply fill a pot with water, and put the chocolate pieces into a bowl that fits securely over the pot. Make sure the water does not touch the bowl. Cook over low heat, stirring, until all the chocolate is melted.

Pour the melted chocolate into the bowl with the almonds. Mix together well with a spoon, so that all the almonds are covered evenly with chocolate. Using a spatula, scoop up the chocolate-covered almonds, and shake off any extra chocolate. Place them on the prepared baking sheet and lightly sprinkle with the cayenne pepper and sea salt. Refrigerate for at least 25 minutes, until the chocolate hardens. You can store in an airtight container in the refrigerator until they're ready to be enjoyed.

SPICED TURMERIC POPCORN

If you haven't started popping your own popcorn yet, today marks the big day. There's no going back to the packaged stuff after you've popped your own. Homemade popcorn is so easy to make, will save you money and is often more nutritious. This spicy garlic turmeric mix complements popcorn beautifully. Turmeric is a medicinal spice rich in curcumin, which has strong anti-inflammatory properties. It lends a rich yellow color to this recipe, and along with the garlic powder and cayenne pepper, adds richness in flavor as well.

Gluten-free / Vegan / 30 minutes or less

Serves: 5
Per Serving / Calories: 140 / **Carbohydrates:** 23 g / **Protein:** 3 g / **Fat:** 4 g

- 1 tbsp (14 g) coconut oil
- ⅔ cup (110 g) popcorn kernels
- 1 tsp turmeric powder
- 1 tsp garlic powder
- Salt and cayenne pepper to taste

Add the coconut oil to a large pot that has a lid. Add one popcorn kernel to the pot, cover it with the lid and place over medium heat. It should take 2 to 3 minutes for that one kernel to pop. When the first kernel pops, add the rest of the popcorn kernels, making sure they are spread out evenly and not piled on top of each other. Replace the lid and cook for 1 minute.

The kernels should have started popping by the end of the 1-minute mark. Now, slightly crack the pot cover to allow some steam to escape without having the popcorn jump out. Let the kernels pop for another 3 minutes.

Meanwhile, combine the turmeric and garlic powder in a small bowl. Pour the popcorn into a large bowl, sprinkle with the spice mix and finish off with salt and cayenne pepper to taste. Mix well.

Store any remaining popcorn in a tightly sealed zip-top bag at room temperature.

PISTACHIO POMEGRANATE YOGURT BARK

We're always looking for new and creative ways to enjoy Greek yogurt. So when we discovered yogurt bark on the Internet, we knew we had to give it a try. In this recipe, we pair two of our favorite foods—pistachios and pomegranates—and enjoy them in this delicious and healthy recipe. Greek yogurt is our yogurt of choice simply because it has half the sugar of traditional yogurt and almost double the protein. One serving of this beauty of a snack will earn you 10 grams of protein, which will help you feel satiated for hours.

Gluten-free

Serves: 2
Per Serving / Calories: 166 / **Carbohydrates:** 18 g / **Protein:** 10 g / **Fat:** 7 g

- 2 tbsp (15 g) shelled pistachios
- ¾ cup (184 g) nonfat vanilla Greek yogurt
- ¼ cup (44 g) pomegranate seeds
- 1 tbsp (20 ml) honey (optional)

Line a baking dish with parchment paper—either a 7 x 11-inch (18 x 28-cm) or 9 x 9-inch (23 x 23-cm) baking dish will do the trick here.

Pour the pistachios into a zip-top bag and crush them with a heavy object. We used a hammer but this is your chance to get creative.

Spread the Greek yogurt across the parchment paper. Sprinkle on the pomegranate seeds and crushed pistachios. Transfer the baking dish to the freezer and freeze for 5 to 6 hours, or until frozen.

When frozen, break the bark into pieces. Have half now and save the rest for later. Remember, this snack must be consumed shortly after you take it out of the freezer, so don't take this with you for an on-the-go snack and expect it to last for hours, as it will melt quickly.

If you want to add the honey, drizzle it on before serving. Note that this will increase the calories by about 30 per serving, and up the carb content by 9 grams.

GRANOLA APPLE CHOCOLATE CHIP "COOKIES"

Okay, so maybe these aren't exactly "cookies," but they are as delicious as cookies. We make this recipe with kids all the time and they always seem to love it. One thing we always mention to our patients is that while granola is technically healthy, it is a high-calorie food (remember, it's oats baked in oil), so we recommend not going overboard with your serving. If we are having granola as part of a snack, we try to keep the granola under ¼ cup (31 g) per serving.

Gluten-free (if using gluten-free granola) / Vegan (if using dark chocolate chips/dairy-free chocolate chips) / 30 minutes or less

Serves: 2
Per Serving / Calories: 183 / **Carbohydrates:** 22 g / **Protein:** 4 g / **Fat:** 14 g

· **1 apple**
· **2 tbsp (32 g) peanut butter**
· **2 tbsp (10 g) granola**
· **2 tbsp (21 g) chocolate chips**

Core the apple, removing the stem and all of the seeds, then slice into six rings. Spread a thin layer of peanut butter on each apple ring, then sprinkle on the granola and chocolate chips. Enjoy!

ZUCCHINI PIZZA BITES

This zucchini "pizza" recipe is unique because there is absolutely no dough involved. It takes all of 5 minutes to prepare and kids love it. Seriously, we make it with our kids' groups and they can't get enough. If making this for children, we keep it basic: only pizza sauce, mozzarella and zucchini. Here, we spice things up a bit to cater to your more sophisticated taste buds. We hope you like!

Gluten-free / 30 minutes or less

Serves: 2
Per Serving / Calories: 120 / **Carbohydrates:** 11 g / **Protein:** 8 g / **Fat:** 5 g

- 1 zucchini
- 5 pitted black olives
- ⅛ red onion
- 5 tsp (25.5 g) pizza sauce
- ⅓ cup (37 g) shredded mozzarella cheese
- 1 tsp Italian seasoning or oregano

Preheat the oven to 375°F (190°C). Line a baking sheet with parchment paper.

Cut the zucchini into rounds that are about ¼ inch (6 mm) thick. Finely dice the olives and red onion.

Add a dab of pizza sauce to each zucchini round, then sprinkle on the mozzarella cheese. Top with the black olives and onion and sprinkle with the Italian seasoning. Place on the prepared baking sheet and bake for 10 to 15 minutes, or until the zucchini is cooked and the cheese is melted.

GARLIC-ROASTED CHICKPEAS

These garlic-roasted chickpeas will provide a savory crunch that will help get you through the week. Chickpeas are insanely delicious and provide an excellent dose of fiber, protein and iron. They are super flexible in the kitchen and can be used for baking, salads, dressings, stews and so much more. The coconut soy sauce drizzled onto the chickpeas before roasting creates a deep brown finish.

Gluten-free (if using gluten-free soy sauce) / Vegan

Serves: 4
Per Serving / Calories: 154 / **Carbohydrates:** 16 g / **Protein:** 5 g / **Fat:** 8 g

- 1 (15.5-oz [358-g]) can chickpeas, drained and rinsed
- 2 tbsp (27 g) coconut oil
- 1 tsp garlic powder
- 1 tsp soy sauce
- Salt and cayenne pepper to taste

Preheat the oven to 400°F (204°C). Line a baking sheet with parchment paper.

Spread the chickpeas on a paper towel. Use another piece of paper towel to pat the chickpeas dry. Allow the chickpeas to air-dry for at least 30 minutes.

In the meantime, combine the coconut oil, garlic powder and soy sauce in a small bowl and stir well.

Spread the dried chickpeas on the prepared baking sheet. Brush the coconut oil spice mix onto the chickpeas, and bake for 35 minutes or until crisp and browned. About 15 minutes into baking, flip the chickpeas so that they cook evenly. Sprinkle with the salt and cayenne pepper to taste. Although this snack is best enjoyed fresh, you can store the chickpeas in an airtight container at room temperature for 2 to 3 days.

UNBAKED COCONUT WALNUT BROWNIES

Unbaked brownies? Yes, you read correctly. These yummy snacks are made with dates and require no oven time. You simply pulse the ingredients together, and in a few easy steps you'll have a sweet and nutritious snack for the week. Besides adding a dose of sweetness, dates provide fiber, potassium and iron. When soaked in water, they develop a soft texture that will help keep the brownies together.

Gluten-free / Vegan

Makes: 8 brownies

Per Serving / Calories: 180 / **Carbohydrates:** 19 g / **Protein:** 4 g / **Fat:** 13 g

- 1 cup (147 g) pitted dates
- 1⅓ cup (155.6 g) chopped walnuts, divided
- ½ cup (43 g) unsweetened cocoa powder
- ¼ cup (23.3 g) unsweetened coconut flakes

Line a baking sheet with parchment paper.

Place the pitted dates in a bowl, cover with warm water and soak for 30 minutes. Drain. Add the dates, 1 cup (117 g) of the walnuts, cocoa powder and coconut flakes to a food processor. Pulse until a consistent, thick paste has formed.

Scoop out the mixture onto the prepared sheet and spread it evenly with a large spoon or spatula, shaping it into a long rectangle about 1 inch (2.5 cm) in height. Press the remaining ⅓ cup (38.6 g) chopped walnuts into the top. Refrigerate for at least an hour.

Cut it into eight squares and store them in an airtight container in the refrigerator for up to 1 week.

CHEWY CRANBERRY ENERGY BALLS

It's Monday. Three o'clock. You had lunch three hours ago and are feeling like you need a pick-me-up. Instead of heading to the vending machine, pull out this snack (you'll have to plan ahead for this, but it's so worth it). We love these energy bites because they're easy, delicious and balanced—everything a nutritionist could ask for in a snack. This recipe is perfect for a reboot because it's full of blood sugar–stabilizing protein from the almonds and peanut butter. The oats give you a dose of complex carbohydrates while the chia seeds provide a serving of omega-3 fatty acids, which are good for the heart.

Gluten-free (if using gluten-free oats) / 30 minutes or less

Serves: 5

Per Serving (2 balls) / **Calories:** 175 / **Carbohydrates:** 18 g / **Protein:** 5 g / **Fat:** 10 g

- ½ cup (41 g) rolled oats
- ¼ cup (40 g) dried cranberries
- ¼ cup (34 g) chopped almonds
- 4 tsp (22 g) peanut butter (almond butter works well here, too)
- 1 tsp honey
- 1 tsp chia seeds

Roll up your sleeves because this one can get messy. Toss all the ingredients into a food processor and pulse until the dough reaches an even, but chunky, consistency. Remove from the food processor and roll the mixture into ten balls. And that's it—they're ready to go. Place the leftovers in an airtight mason jar or a container in the fridge for up to 1 week for optimal storage.

QUENCH YOUR THIRST WITH THESE REFRESHING, HEALTHY BEVERAGES

We get it. Water can get a little dull sometimes, which is why we whipped up six alternatives to keep you hydrated and feeling good. With sugary beverages made readily available everywhere, it's important to avoid drinking your calories when possible. Thirst quenchers like our Rosemary Green Tea Limeade and Basil Watermelon Spritzer (page 208) provide a touch of sweetness without the excessive sugar and calories. Our drink recipes come packed with a range of antioxidants, vitamins and minerals. If you're being mindful of calories, be sure to factor these drinks into your daily intake.

ROSEMARY GREEN TEA LIMEADE

Rosemary is a highly aromatic herb and it perfectly complements the flavors in green tea. The maple syrup brings out the sweet, earthy tones of this herb, and the result is a comforting beverage with citrus, spice and everything nice. We are both huge fans of green tea because of its affordability and the endless nutritional benefits it provides. It is loaded with antioxidants, and recent studies have shown that it has the potential to yield positive effects for weight loss, diabetes and heart disease.

Gluten-free / Vegan / 30 minutes or less

Serves: 3
Per Serving / Calories: 42 **/ Carbohydrates:** 11 g **/ Protein:** 0 g **/ Fat:** 0 g

- 6 cups (1.4 L) water
- 2 sprigs fresh rosemary
- 3 bags green tea
- 1 lime
- 2 tbsp (30 ml) maple syrup

In a pot, bring the water to a boil over high heat. Then add the fresh rosemary, and boil for 5 minutes. Remove the pot from the stove, and steep the green tea bags in the rosemary water for 3 minutes, dunking the bags in and out a few times. Discard the tea bags and allow the rosemary tea water to cool. Squeeze the lime juice into the pot, and stir in the maple syrup for sweetness, mixing well using a large spoon. Finish off with ice cubes if you prefer a cooler drink.

EASY MATCHA LATTE

When this green tea first came on the foodie scene a year or two ago, we weren't sure what all the fuss was about. Then we did our research and quickly realized that this superfood deserves the hype. Just for a little background, matcha is made from shade-grown leaves and literally means "powdered tea." Because matcha is derived from ground tea leaves, the antioxidant properties are higher. Some studies suggest that the polyphenols found in matcha are linked to protection against cancer and heart disease, blood sugar control and antiaging. Ready to give this a try?

Gluten-free / 30 minutes or less

Serves: 1 / **Calories:** 87 / **Carbohydrates:** 9 g / **Protein:** 2 g / **Fat:** 5 g

- 1½ cups (360 ml) unsweetened almond milk
- 1 tsp matcha powder
- 1 tsp honey

In a small pot, bring the almond milk to a simmer over medium-high heat until the milk is hot. While this is heating, add the matcha powder to a glass or ceramic cup. Slowly whisk in the hot almond milk (about ¼ cup [60 ml] at a time) until the matcha powder dissolves. If you hold the cup at an angle as you pour the milk, you'll create more foam to add more of a "latte" effect. Stir in the honey to sweeten.

ANTIOXIDANT GREEN SMOOTHIE

There are two types of smoothies: snack smoothies and meal smoothies. A meal smoothie (that you would have for, say, breakfast) should include vegetables, fruit, protein and healthy fats. A snack smoothie, on the other hand, doesn't need to be as dense. In fact, because we recommend keeping snacks to less than 200 calories per serving, you want to add a little bit less ingredients to a snack smoothie so you don't overdo the calories. This simple green smoothie is one of our favorite recipes because it's so easy to make. We have it every night an hour or two after dinner to refresh our bodies and press "control-alt-delete" on those after-dinner munchies. Best of all, it's an easy way to consume 3 cups (680 g) of vegetables without even trying. Thirsty? Why wait?

Gluten-free / Vegan / 30 minutes or less

Serves: 1 (Chia seeds not used in calculation) **/ Calories:** 150 **/ Carbohydrates:** 26 g **/ Protein:** 5 g **/ Fat:** 4 g

- 1 cup (240 ml) unsweetened almond milk
- ½ green apple
- ½ cucumber
- 1 stalk celery
- 2 cups (60 g) raw spinach
- 1 small bunch cilantro
- Juice of 1 lime
- 1 tsp chia seeds (optional)
- ½ cup (70 g) ice cubes

Add the almond milk to a high-speed blender. Then add the apple, cucumber, celery, spinach, cilantro, lime juice and chia seeds. Add the ice and blend until smooth.

SPICED CASHEW MILK

The secret to this recipe is homemade cashew milk. because it's extra thick and creamy. If you have a high-speed blender, you can make homemade cashew milk very easily by soaking 1 cup [137 g] of cashews in 4 cups (946 ml) of water for 4 hours. then blending until creamy. If you don't have a high-speed blender handy, that's okay, too—just make this recipe, which simply involves one extra step.

Gluten-free / Vegan

Serves: 4

Per Serving / Calories: 174 / **Carbohydrates:** 9 g / **Protein:** 5 g / **Fat:** 13 g

HOMEMADE CASHEW MILK

- 1 cup (137 g) raw unsalted cashews
- 7 cups (1.7 L) water, divided

SPICED CASHEW MILK

- 7 cups (1.7 L) homemade cashew milk
- ½ cup (70 g) ice cubes
- 1 tsp stevia
- 1 tsp ground nutmeg
- 1 tsp ground cinnamon
- 1 tsp vanilla extract
- 1 tsp ground cloves (optional)
- 1 cinnamon stick (optional, for garnish)

For the cashew milk, soak the cashews in 4 cups (946 ml) of the water for 3 to 4 hours. Drain. In a blender, blend the cashews with the remaining 3 cups (710 ml) of fresh water until smooth. Pour the liquid through a cheesecloth or a fine-mesh strainer into a bowl. That's it.

For the spiced cashew milk, blend the cashew milk. ice cubes, stevia, nutmeg, cinnamon, vanilla and cloves. Blend and add an optional cinnamon stick for garnish. Enjoy!

BASIL WATERMELON SPRITZER

This hydrating watermelon spritzer is simple and refreshing. The aromatic fresh basil works beautifully to bring out the subtle sweetness of the watermelon. Besides being insanely delicious, watermelon happens to be a nutritional superstar. It contains high levels of vitamins A and C, and it is one of the few foods that contains a large amount of lycopene, a powerful antioxidant that helps give watermelon its bright red color.

Gluten-free / Vegan / 30 minutes or less

Serves: 2
Per Serving / Calories: 60 / **Carbohydrates:** 16 g / **Protein:** 1 g / **Fat:** 0 g

· **3 cups (462 g) cubed watermelon**
· **1 tbsp (3 g) chopped fresh basil**
· **½ cup (118 ml) seltzer water**
· **8 ice cubes**
· **Basil leaves, for garnish (optional)**

In a blender, combine the watermelon and basil leaves and blend until smooth. Pour it through a fine-mesh strainer over a bowl and press on the mixture until all of the liquid has been extracted and pressed from the watermelon flesh. Pour the watermelon basil juice into 2 glasses, add ¼ (60 ml) cup seltzer water to each glass, and add four of the ice cubes to each glass to chill. Garnish with fresh basil for a fun finishing touch!

CITRUS GRAPEFRUIT SELTZER

Looking for a dose of flavor and vitamin C? We've got you covered. This citrus seltzer is great for those hotter months, when you're looking to chill out and cool down. Both grapefruit and strawberries provide a strong dose of antioxidants, which have been shown to decrease oxidative damage to body tissues. These fruits, paired with lemon, basil and maple syrup, make for an absolutely delicious concoction.

Gluten-free / Vegan / 30 minutes or less

Serves: 4

Per Serving / **Calories:** 61 / **Carbohydrates:** 16 g / **Protein:** 1 g / **Fat:** 0 g

- 1 qt (946 ml) seltzer water
- Juice of 1 medium grapefruit
- Juice of ½ lemon
- 4 strawberries, sliced
- 2 tbsp (30 ml) maple syrup
- 4 fresh basil leaves

Pour the seltzer water into a large jar or pitcher. Squeeze the grapefruit and lemon juices into the seltzer. Add the sliced strawberries and maple syrup. Using a large spoon, stir to make sure the sweetness is distributed throughout. Garnish with the fresh basil, and allow the flavors to infuse for at least 15 minutes. Pour into a glass and enjoy!

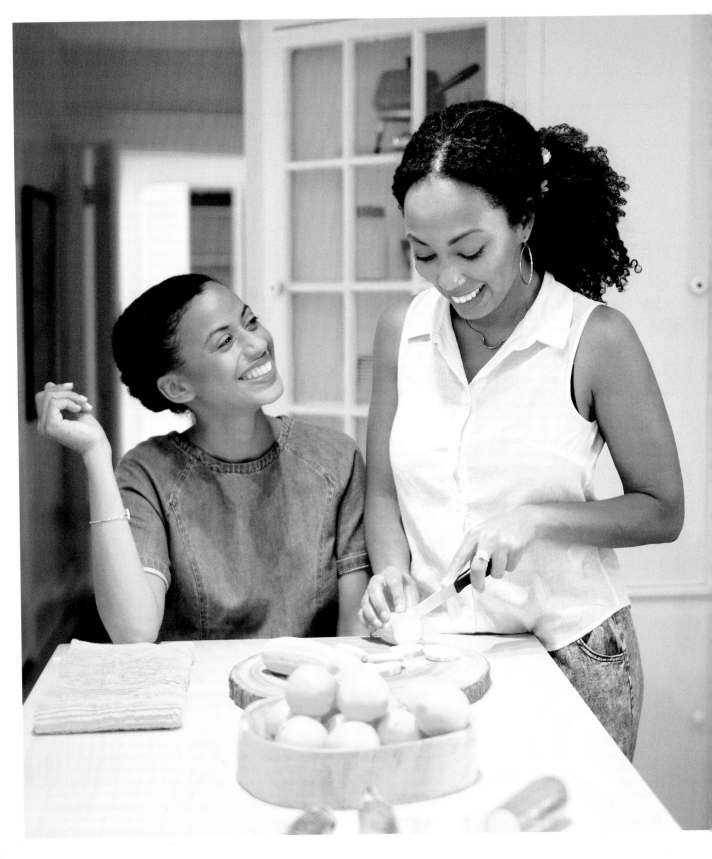

PART 4

Creating Healthy Habits That Last

You've been eating wholesome plant-based foods for the past 28 days, and now it's time to develop the skills you've learned in the kitchen into a lifestyle that sticks. Building new habits isn't the easiest thing to do, and there are many challenges you may come across. Although maintaining consistency can be tricky, it is definitely achievable. Enjoy the process of living a healthier, more balanced lifestyle, and know that it's absolutely okay to have slips. Even as dietitians, we don't have it all figured out, and it can sometimes takes great intention and motivation to maintain these healthy habits.

Start by identifying your motivators for eating healthy, plant-based meals. You may be interested in preventing or managing chronic health conditions. You may want to improve your energy levels, lose weight or set a positive example for your family. It's important to take a moment and think about the different motivators that will push you into sustaining positive lifestyle changes.

Once your motivators have been identified, set measurable and realistic goals. Research suggests that creating small, yet realistic goals when it comes to healthy eating is an excellent way to stay on track. Perhaps after reading this book, you're ready to make the full transition into becoming a vegetarian. Perhaps you're not ready or don't want to be a vegetarian, but you want to incorporate plant-based eating into your lifestyle. Either way is completely fine! Develop measurable goals that will promote healthier dietary habits and reflect the kinds of changes you are ready to make. The following are some examples of goals you can set:

- ☐ I will eat 3 cups (680 g) of vegetables every day.
- ☐ I will prepare at least four vegetarian meals per week.
- ☐ I will stop drinking sugary juices and sodas and will opt for healthier alternatives.

Try not to be hard on yourself and guilt-trip over slip-ups. We actually encourage you to occasionally indulge in your favorite (not-so-healthy) treats. When you've developed a strong foundation for healthy lifestyle changes, those chocolate chip cookies are really not going to kill you. However, try not to have your kitchen stocked with tempting treats that will make overindulging more likely to happen.

Find support in friends, family, colleagues and online. Tap into resources that will keep you motivated. You shouldn't have to do this alone, and there are many people out there who are going through a similar process and want support as well.

Lastly, make this process as fun as possible, keeping in mind that challenges will present themselves. It's all about how you handle them.

ESSENTIAL KITCHEN TOOLS

Equipping your kitchen with certain tools will make cooking so much easier. We both live in really small apartments and prefer to stick to the basics rather than getting a wide range of kitchen gadgets that take up space and cost a fortune. This guide is especially useful for those who are new to cooking and want to learn exactly where to start with healthy eating. Below is a list of kitchen essentials that will get you through this reboot and a lifetime of healthy eating to come. We encourage you to add your favorites to this list, improvise with what you already have and get creative!

BAKING DISH

Have at least one of these in the kitchen for preparing baked dishes, like our Vegetable Layered Lasagna (page 111). We typically use ceramic baking dishes, but you can also use glass or metal. Although you can invest in different sizes, if purchasing just one, go for a medium-sized dish (8 x 8 inch [20.5 x 20.5 cm]).

BAKING SHEET

Baking sheets are flat pans that are typically used for foods like pizzas, cookies and pastries. We prefer stainless steel baking sheets and usually line them with parchment paper for minimal cleanup after cooking.

BLENDER

The blender is hands down one of our favorite kitchen tools. You throw everything in there and a few seconds later you have a consistent batch of heavenly goodness. A good blender can be used for smoothies, soups, batters, dressings and more. We each have a personal-size blender and full-size high-speed blender in our kitchens. When making single-serving smoothies, it's easier to work with the personal-size blender. For soups and batters, the full-size blender is more appropriate.

BOWLS

When preparing recipes, bowls are great for organizing ingredients. They're also perfect for marinating and mixing things like salads and batters. We suggest you invest in at least four bowls ranging in size from small to large. We typically use stainless steel. Other options include glass, wood and ceramic.

CAST-IRON SKILLET

Cast-iron skillets can be used for baking, grilling and cooking on gas or electric stove tops. They can sustain temperatures up to 500°F (260°C) and are extremely flexible in the kitchen. It's one of our most-used kitchen tools, and as long as you maintain it properly, it can last you a lifetime. To clean your skillet, wash it by hand using hot water and a sponge. Avoid soaking or using soap or steel wool. Towel dry the skillet and dry it on the stove over low heat. Then apply vegetable oil to a paper towel and rub it on the inside and outside of the skillet to prevent rusting.

CUTTING BOARD

It's a good idea to have three different cutting boards in your kitchen: a small one, for chopping smaller foods like garlic, tomatoes and onions; a medium-sized board for slicing foods like plantains, potatoes, eggplant and other larger foods; and a larger board for any animal products you might be preparing. For the meat, poultry and seafood eaters among us, we definitely suggest you invest in a separate cutting board to avoid cross-contamination. Make sure you wash the boards thoroughly in hot, soapy water after each use.

ELECTRIC GRILL PRESS

This is another favorite that proves to be particularly useful in making quesadillas, grilled cheeses and veggie burgers. You can just pop your assembled meal into the press, and five minutes later, it's ready to enjoy.

FOOD PROCESSOR

Food processors are great for creating a consistent mix of ingredients and are especially useful when making spreads and dips. Blenders usually require some liquid for mixing to happen, whereas food processors don't need any. They make food prep so much easier and cut down on time spent in the kitchen.

HAND MIXER

Hand mixers are great for beating, whipping and mixing. They are pretty affordable and don't require much maintenance. If you're looking to get a good arm workout, opt for a whisk. If you're like us and prefer the shortcut, buy a hand mixer.

KNIFE SET

Invest in a good knife set that includes a chef's knife, a paring knife and a serrated utility knife. Many knife sets come equipped with a knife sharpener, which you should use to keep your knives in top condition. We use a stainless steel set that comes equipped with a range of small, medium and large knives.

LARGE SPOONS

Have at least two large cooking spoons for mixing and stirring. In our kitchens, we use stainless steel, bamboo and wooden spoons.

LOAF PAN

Loaf pans are useful for making all types of breads. In this book, we feature a delicious Banana Blueberry Bread (page 35), which is made in a stainless steel mini-loaf pan. If making larger batches of breads, opt for a 3- or 4-cup (8 x 4-inch [20.5 x 10-cm]) loaf pan.

MASON JARS

We use mason jars for pretty much everything—storing food, packing lunch, serving drinks, you name it. They're so useful and can be purchased for a reasonable price.

MUFFIN PAN

We use nonstick 6-cup muffin pans for our recipes. If needed, adjust the baking time for smaller pans. Muffin pans are also great for freezing leftover soups, stews and sauces.

OIL MISTER

Oil misters provide a fine, even spray of oil to your pots and pans. This prevents foods sticking to the bottom and lets you better control the amount of calories in your dishes. You can purchase an actual oil mister or get a regular spray bottle and fill it with your favorite cooking oil.

PARCHMENT PAPER

Parchment paper is typically used for baking and provides a nonstick surface that can be easily disposed of when you're finished cooking. We usually line baking sheets with parchment paper to minimize cleanup.

PEELER

A peeler can be used to remove the skin from fruits and vegetables. You can also use it to shave cheese, zest citrus or create vegetable strips. We prefer a Y-head peeler, which is inexpensive and easy to use.

POTS AND PANS

The options out there for pots and pans can be overwhelming, so we'll stick to the basics. Invest in a saucepan, a sauté pan, a frying pan and a stockpot. The sizes should reflect how many people you usually cook for, although we recommend you have a range of small to medium-sized pots and pans. Most of your pots and pans should come with lids, as you will sometimes use them during the cooking process.

SPATULA

Although we usually use spatulas for flipping, they can also be used for spreading and lifting. We typically use a metal spatula for our recipes.

SPIRALIZER

Spiralizers are such a fun, inexpensive tool! They can be used to make noodles out of various vegetables, and they add a creative twist to plant-based recipes.

STORAGE CONTAINERS

It's so important to have quality containers that will properly store your food, both in the refrigerator and when you pack it for on-the-go meals and snacks. Buy a container set with options for storing soups, salads, larger meals and dressings. We typically use glass jars and glass containers with locking lids.

WHISK

If you don't have a hand mixer, or don't want to take it out, a whisk is helpful for whipping up ingredients. We use a metal balloon whisk.

STOCK YOUR PANTRY

Having a pantry stocked with essentials makes the process of cooking so much easier. Instead of having to purchase things like oils, spices and flavor enhancers each time you go to the supermarket, you'll already have them ready to go. We compiled a Food Heaven Pantry List, which reflects all of the essential pantry ingredients we use throughout this book. We recommend that you take a look in your cabinets and mark off which ingredients you have and which ones you need to purchase. There may be some spices, oils or other essentials that you absolutely cannot live without. We encourage you to add them to this list and incorporate them into recipes as you see fit.

- ☐ Apple cider vinegar
- ☐ Baking powder
- ☐ Baking soda
- ☐ Balsamic vinegar
- ☐ Bay leaves
- ☐ Black pepper
- ☐ Brown sugar
- ☐ Canola oil
- ☐ Cayenne pepper
- ☐ Chia seeds
- ☐ Chili powder
- ☐ Coconut oil
- ☐ Cornstarch
- ☐ Crushed red pepper flakes

- ☐ Curry powder
- ☐ Garlic powder
- ☐ Ground cinnamon
- ☐ Ground cumin
- ☐ Ground flaxseed
- ☐ Ground nutmeg
- ☐ Liquid stevia
- ☐ Maple syrup
- ☐ Nutritional yeast
- ☐ Olive oil
- ☐ Onion powder
- ☐ Oregano
- ☐ Paprika
- ☐ Red cooking wine

- ☐ Rice vinegar
- ☐ Salt
- ☐ Sesame seed oil
- ☐ Smoked paprika
- ☐ Soy sauce or Bragg's liquid aminos
- ☐ Sriracha sauce
- ☐ Stevia
- ☐ Unsweetened cocoa powder
- ☐ Unsweetened coconut flakes
- ☐ Vanilla extract
- ☐ Vegetable oil

WEEK 2 MEAL PLANNING CHART

DAY	BREAKFAST	LUNCH	DINNER	SNACKS
SUNDAY				
MONDAY				
TUESDAY				
WEDNESDAY				
THURSDAY				
FRIDAY				
SATURDAY				

SAMPLE GROCERY LIST

FRUITS	VEGETABLES	HERBS	GRAINS	BEANS	NUTS AND SEEDS	EGGS AND DAIRY	PANTRY ITEMS	OTHER

*Don't forget to create a shopping list and organize your recipes so they are ready to go.
Wash fruit, chop veggies and organize snacks.

WEEK 3 MEAL PLANNING CHART

DAY	BREAKFAST	LUNCH	DINNER	SNACKS
SUNDAY				
MONDAY				
TUESDAY				
WEDNESDAY				
THURSDAY				
FRIDAY				
SATURDAY				

SAMPLE GROCERY LIST

FRUITS	VEGETABLES	HERBS	GRAINS	BEANS	NUTS AND SEEDS	EGGS AND DAIRY	PANTRY ITEMS	OTHER

Don't forget to create a shopping list and organize your recipes so they are ready to go.
Wash fruit, chop veggies and organize snacks.

WEEK 4 MEAL PLANNING CHART

DAY	BREAKFAST	LUNCH	DINNER	SNACKS
SUNDAY				
MONDAY				
TUESDAY				
WEDNESDAY				
THURSDAY				
FRIDAY				
SATURDAY				

SAMPLE GROCERY LIST

FRUITS	VEGETABLES	HERBS	GRAINS	BEANS	NUTS AND SEEDS	EGGS AND DAIRY	PANTRY ITEMS	OTHER

*Don't forget to create a shopping list and organize your recipes so they are ready to go. Wash fruit, chop veggies and organize snacks.

ACKNOWLEDGMENTS

We are eternally grateful for all of the love, support and guidance we've received in creating this book. There are so many people we have come across who helped spark our creativity and inspired us, and we can't even begin to express how thankful we are. Our patients continue to be the driving force behind our creation of nutrition-focused tools and resources. Thank you for allowing us to work with you. Throughout the years, we've been able to listen to your stories, challenges and successes. All of your insight has inspired us to not only create this book, but to also actively explore other creative ways of making food enjoyable and nourishing.

Thank you to our colleagues and professors, who have mentored us, and continue to provide a constant source of support and knowledge. Thank you to our tribe of friends and family, for always being down to taste our recipes and flesh out ideas. Your honest and useful feedback has been invaluable. A big shout out to our parents: They had a major influence on many of the recipes in this book, and worked with us every step of the way to make sure the meals created met their very high standards. We'd also like to thank our sisters for their amazing support and stamp of approval on the photographs and cover shot selection. Thank you to our community of readers over at Food Heaven Made Easy. We started our brand more than 5 years ago and can't believe how much we've been able to accomplish. Your comments, emails and messages give us life, and we are so excited to continue this journey with you.

A special thank you to our photographer extraordinaire, Toni Zernik. Your passion for food and photography shines radiantly in this book. Thank you for allowing us to crash your home, bounce ideas off of you and create a work of art. We'd also like to thank our freelance nutrition consultant Maggie DePiero, who put in countless hours creating the nutrition facts for all of these recipes, and helped us curate the sample 1-week meal plan and grocery list we provide in the beginning of this book. We'd also like to thank our interns for your help in the fact-checking process.

A big thank you to our publisher, for believing in our vision and making this book a reality. This is a dream come true for us and we truly appreciate your support throughout every step of the process.

ABOUT THE AUTHORS

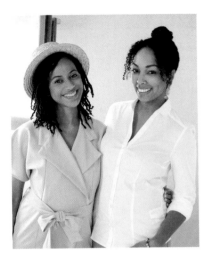

Jessica Jones, MS, RDN, CDE, is an outpatient Registered Dietitian/Nutritionist at a community clinic in Oakland, California. As a Registered Dietitian and Certified Diabetes Educator with a certificate of training in adult weight management, Jessica counsels hundreds of clients on weight management, pre-diabetes/diabetes, high cholesterol, hypertension, GI issues, wellness and vegan/vegetarian nutrition. She also teaches weekly classes in both English and Spanish on diabetes prevention and healthy living for kids and families. In addition to her love of hands-on nutrition education and counseling, Jessica has a passion for using media as a tool to promote healthy lifestyles. With a B.A. in Journalism from San Francisco State University, Jones has penned hundreds of articles about food, health and culture for publications like *Time Out New York*, Buzzfeed, Self.com, and *Today's Dietitian*.

Wendy Lopez, MS, RDN, is a Registered Dietitian/Nutritionist who is passionate about educating communities on plant-based eating, in ways that are accessible and culturally relevant. Working as a clinical dietitian in a community clinic in Port Chester, New York, Wendy focuses on disease prevention and management. She uses an integrative and individualized approach toward nutrition, health and well-being. Wendy was raised in the Bronx, with roots in the Dominican Republic. When not catching up on the latest nutrition science, you can find her cooking, traveling, basking in the sun and obsessively working on home improvement projects.

FOR MORE ON WENDY AND JESS, VISIT WWW.FOODHEAVENMADEEASY.COM

INDEX